# SPEECH DISORDERS

*Founded by C. K. Ogden*

# The International Library of Psychology

## COGNITIVE PSYCHOLOGY
### In 21 Volumes

# SPEECH DISORDERS

## A Psychological Study of the Various Defects of Speech

SARA M STINCHFIELD

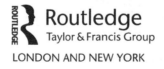

Routledge
Taylor & Francis Group

LONDON AND NEW YORK

First published in 1933 by
Routledge, Trench, Trubner & Co., Ltd.
2 Park Square, Milton Park, Abingdon, Oxfordshire OX14 4RN
711 Third Avenue, New York, NY 10017

First issued in paperback 2014

*Routledge is an imprint of the Taylor and Francis Group, an informa business*

© 1933 Sara M Stinchfield

*British Library Cataloguing in Publication Data*
A CIP catalogue record for this book
is available from the British Library

Speech Disorders
ISBN 0415-20975-7
Cognitive Psychology: 21 Volumes
ISBN 0415-21126-3
The International Library of Psychology: 204 Volumes
ISBN 0415-19132-7

ISBN 13: 978-1-138-87508-1 (pbk)
ISBN 13: 978-0-415-20975-5 (hbk)

To

MY FORMER COLLEAGUES

IN THE DEPARTMENT OF PSYCHOLOGY

MOUNT HOLYOKE COLLEGE

ELLEN BLISS TALBOT

AND

SAMUEL PERKINS HAYES

# PREFACE

RECENT surveys made by clinical workers in public schools and in university centres seem to indicate that speech disorders are on the increase, and that additional facilities are needed for dealing with the speech-handicapped child or adolescent, because of the bearing of speech disorders upon personality, socialization and economic success.

The findings of the White House Conference Committee, as reported by Drs. Travis and West, and Miss Camp, indicated that there are at least a million children with speech defects in the United States. Children with speech handicaps are being referred to child guidance and hospital clinics with increasing frequency, and the writer offers this volume hoping that it may be of service to the speech-pathologist, laliatrist, speech clinical worker, teacher of speech correction, case worker, physician or psychiatrist to whom such cases are referred.

The writer wishes to express her appreciation to the following friends who have made valuable suggestions regarding certain chapters : to the late Dr. Theodore Hoch, Northampton State Hospital ; Dr. R. N. Hat, Springfield Shriner's Hospital ; to my former colleague, Dr. Herbert Moore, and to Dr. Grace Fernald of University of California at Los Angeles, for suggestions on the chapter on Oral and Silent Reading ; and suggestions received from my colleague Dr. Milton K. Metfessel ; to Dr. Robert Wälder of Vienna and to Dr. Shepard I. Franz for suggestions regarding the chapter on Dysphasia ; to Miss Eileen MacLeod, King's College Hospital, London, and to Prof. Lloyd James, School of Oriental Studies, London, for suggestions regarding phonetic defects and difficulties ; to Dr. Emil Fröschels, Speech Clinic, University of Vienna, for valuable suggestions, theories and

training given in the field of speech pathology ; to Miss
Lucile McLaughlin, psychology major at Mount Holyoke
College, for assistance in tabulations made for the chapter
on Speech Data ; to my colleagues at Mount Holyoke
College in the departments of Psychology, Speech, Health,
Physical Education and Physiology, for assistance in
securing data ; to Dr. and Mrs. S. P. Hayes for their
careful reading and corrections on the entire manuscript ;
to Samuel D. Robbins, chairman of the terminology
committee for the American Society for the Study of
Disorders of Speech, for permission to use the published
and unpublished classifications of speech disorders on
which we have worked jointly ; for the excellent studies
of cleft-palatal cases the writer wishes to express her
indebtedness to Dr. J. J. Fitzgibbon, who kindly furnished
the cuts and photographs used in the chapter on cleft-
palate speech ; to my husband, Dr. Charles Lyle Hawk,
for his indefatigable patience and enthusiasm in reading
and correcting manuscript, for the many suggestions
given during its preparation, for furnishing the cuts used
in various chapters, and drawing the bar-graphs in the
chapter on Oral and Silent Reading ; lastly to my mother
for proof-reading copies of various chapters.

SARA M. STINCHFIELD

(Mrs C. L. HAWK).

Los Angeles, California
*November* 1932

# CONTENTS

## PART I

## THE NATURE OF SPEECH DISORDERS

# LIST OF ILLUSTRATIONS

PAGE

TEXT FIGURES

# Part I

## THE NATURE OF SPEECH DISORDERS

Part I

# CHAPTER I

## SPEECH OF INFANCY AND EARLY CHILDHOOD

### (a) NORMAL SPEECH DEVELOPMENT
### (b) ABNORMAL SPEECH DEVELOPMENT

*What Happens when Speech " goes Wrong " ?*

STUDENTS of child psychology, parents, teachers and clinicians, are increasingly interested to know what is happening when a child fails to develop speech at the usual time. Workers with speech-handicapped children recognize the fact that a child is often doubly unfortunate, not only because he possesses a speech peculiarity which sets him somewhat apart from the group, but also because the possession of such a difficulty tends to breed a much more serious concomitant—that of a warped, unsocial or peculiar personality.

We learn from child psychology that long before the child is ready to enter school, his personality is already more or less " set ", determined in certain attitudes or trends, and biased for better or for worse, according to the child's outlook on life and his social environment. If his childhood is the product of what we call a " balanced " home environment, society will be the richer, and may take especial pains to furnish the child with such tools as are needed for fostering his particular abilities.

The problem of the education of the specially-handicapped child is much more difficult however. Here we may find not only a double but even a triple handicap. The child may not only be deaf, but may possess some other handicap besides his speech impediment. He may have other physical or mental defects in addition to deafness. Matters are then more complicated, because

3

we not only have to deal with the child's deafness, blindness, or crippled condition, but we must also bear in mind that he has a speech handicap which distinctly limits his possibilities of attainment. Moreover, along with his special handicap may go personal idiosyncrasies, such as tics, facial grimaces, various mannerisms and little defects of personality which are closely bound up with his physical or mental handicap as well as with his speech difficulty.

In order to consider more carefully the nature and causes of some of the speech disturbances which accompany various special defects such as deafness, blindness, crippled condition, mental deficiency and sub-normality, let us go back to the beginnings of speech in infancy. By recalling some of the facts which have been observed by students of primitive language, and of the origins of speech in babyhood, we may find significant facts which bear upon the problem of how normal speech begins. We may also discover some of the things which happen when normal speech fails to appear.

### Animal Language and Human Speech

Language is defined as a mode of behaviour. A vocal language is found in animals, but this is not identical with the articulate speech of man. The animal gives expression to emotional cries, primitive sounds connected with the immediate moment and with local conditions. Long and patient training of animals such as the chimpanzee and other anthropoids fails to reveal any special aptitude for performing the delicate sequence of muscle, tongue, lip, jaw, soft-palate and vocal-cord activity necessary to produce the articulate speech sounds which begin to appear very early in the human infant. The animal possesses the necessary structures, but lacks the finer control of minute accessory muscles controlling the speech apparatus. His brain does not function on so complex a level as does the human brain. From the fourth month onward the baby may be expected to

make random, spontaneous speech sounds which are very
like the vowels and consonants found in articulate speech.
He does this with no conception of their meaning, and
cannot even reproduce them volitionally, but he is using
some of the finer co-ordinations of the speech organs in
his spontaneous babbling, while the animal infant shows
no such tendency.

Not only do animals use the language of emotion, but
they use some gesture or pantomime which corresponds
roughly to what we find in primitive human society.  If
the animal's vocabulary of expression is chiefly limited
to emotional cries such as groans, grunts, screams, calls,
laughing, clucking, and croons of contentment, we know
that normally the human infant very early develops all
these, and soon shows the ability to emit an additional
series of sounds by means of the movements of special
accessory muscles involved in articulate speech.  Due to
auditory stimuli primarily, and with visual aid or observation, the normal child shows himself to be adept at
imitative movements with these organs long before he
has begun to associate them with definite meanings.[1]
And so we find that the human infant shows a special
aptitude for making these sounds in a non-purposive
way, whereas the various domestic or wild animals under
observation have shown fewer such tendencies.  According
to Negus [2] the use of intelligence is an essential for any
elaboration of the vocal cord, but acquisition of the
powers of vocal communication have given a great spur
to the development of higher intelligence, as in man.

### The Difference a Qualitative One

Microscopic examination of the brain structure of the
anthropoids as compared with man has not revealed any
marked differences, but that there is a qualitative difference is evident from the speed with which the human
infant with a normal brain develops finer accessory
movements.  Animals in the same environment, stimulated

[1] Paget, Sir R., *Babel*, 1930, p. 93.
[2] Negus, V. E., *The Mechanism of the Larynx*, 1929, pp. 309–343.

by the same auditory stimuli, show no such tendencies, and do not even respond to intensive training, except in rare instances, and after a long and tedious process, during which they fail to achieve what the human infant accomplishes in a very short time. Man's greater dexterity in manual movements, in co-ordinations of eye-hand-tongue motions and frequency of practice has led to higher cerebral development and to the attainment of higher skills than the animal possesses.

The dominance-by-brain gives man the advantage over animals of greater size and strength, and accounts for gradations of mental development within the human race, so that we often find dominance of one man or race by another.

The possession of speech skill sets man apart from all other creatures, and renders him the most interesting, the most powerful, the most creative of all, as well as perhaps the most unpredictable and baffling. The way in which man uses this power to dominate, to subjugate, to control, to defend or to barter, and the degree of correspondence between his words and his actions, may make or mar not only interrelations between individuals, but international relations as well, and therefore the psychology of language becomes not merely an interesting object of study and research, but may have a great deal to do with altering geographical and national barriers, or raising barriers where none have formerly existed. It is even contended by international experts that the absence of a common language is the chief obstacle to the progress of international understanding, and therefore the chief underlying cause of war.[1]

Primitive tribes regarded speech symbols of more civilized tribes as a sort of magic, a form of communication mixed with sorcery and black art. A stranger who could not speak the language of a savage tribe was usually regarded as a natural enemy.[2]

---

[1] Ogden, C. K., *Debabelization*, 1931, p. 13.
[2] Malinowski, B., *The Problem of Meaning in Primitive Language*, pp. 451–510.

Speech is the most serviceable way of making ourselves understood, of conveying our wishes accurately, or recording for future use those ideas and ideals which we wish to preserve, through the use of written signs or symbols. If the mental processes which govern language are imperfect, then our thought processes are disorganized and our reasoning power is greatly diminished. If for any reason the language which we use is chaotic, then our social life is at once crippled, while the communication of thought and even of clear thinking, becomes unnecessarily difficult.[1]

### Linguistic Ability of Infants as Compared with Adults

Those who have watched the speech development of the normal infant envy him his linguistic ability, because he acquires a vocabulary which is quite adequate to his needs and to his environment, within a remarkably short space of time. As adults some of us have struggled for years to attain even a mediocre vocabulary in a foreign tongue, and yet we are rarely able to obscure some traces of foreign accent in the new language. The child is bothered by no such difficulty. He babbles and produces random speech sounds similar to those in the language which he hears about him, and reproduces them with surprising accuracy even before he has learned to attach meanings to them. It is said that Belgian refugee children, following the World War, were very soon able to speak the language of their new homes as well as the children who had always spoken it.

Even when various teachers of foreign languages attempt to instruct by the " natural method ", we find that it seems to be impossible to give the essentials to a mixed group of adults within a very brief period, because the situation is artificial, and cannot take the place of the actual situation which surrounds the child who is learning to speak a new language.

[1] Paget, Sir R., *Babel*, p. 11.

## Habit Formation in Speech

If adults are found to be slower than children in acquiring new and perfectly normal speech habits, it is also true that if unfortunate speech habits have been acquired during the speech-learning process, and if they have persisted into adulthood, they will be much harder to displace and to replace with the correct speech habits, than would have been the case in childhood.

Even though a child may show a natural gift for language above that of other children of the same family or neighbourhood, we have no way of making certain that he will learn to make all the speech sounds correctly, or even intelligibly. The chances are that he will give as good sounds as he hears about him, but individual peculiarities, organic or psychic conditions which are unfavourable to normal development, may cause a handicap to occur at any one of a number of stages of growth in speech, as in physical development. As adults we are inclined to take too much for granted in regard to the development of this highly-complex function called " learning to talk ". We forget many of its *drawbacks*, and some of its possible *setbacks*.

## Social Significance of Speech

The social value of speech is so apparent to the "normal" child in a " normal " environment, that he soon learns to make little gestures or signs, even before he can use articulate speech. The sign of negation, for instance, which may at first merely have been a head-movement, to refuse undesired food, soon means " no ", and definite refusal is implied by the turning away of the head. From the earliest months we find that the hand and mouth are closely allied, and along with other motor movements we find the child using considerable tongue activity, as though this were an aid to the acquisition of manual dexterity and motor controls, as in learning to walk.

When the writer's small niece was learning to walk,

she worked so hard to secure balance, that her little body stiffened and straightened into all sorts of chaotic and inco-ordinate movements of trunk, head, and legs before she was able to stand alone or to go forward. Along with this effort went the protrusion of the tongue to one side, and this tongue activity persisted well into the period of gaining muscle control. Another little friend, on beginning to write, worked with great effort at " drawing " the letters, and along with this went the active use of the tongue and its protrusion. Many activities may accompany the gaining of control of the finer accessory muscles, quite normally, and yet disappear, once the desired motor movement for the particular activity has become habitual. Occasionally some such movement becomes " set " or remains as a " tic ", or purposeless muscle movement. This may occur if anything happens to interfere with the child's normal progress at this stage, or if ridicule, imitation by adults or other children, or nervous tension, unduly impresses these accessory movements upon the child's consciousness.[1]

The nervous energy required for the speech-learning process is far greater than the average adult realizes. The infant's crowing and babbling is so spontaneous and seems so enjoyable a performance that we are not accustomed to think of it in the light of calories consumed, or fatiguability of the child. The physiologist has shown us by means of electrical currents, the number of shocks which the neurone of the infant can stand as compared with that of the adult, and we know that the baby can stand less than one-fourth as many shocks per second as the adult, before the nerve becomes fatigued. We know little about the energy requirements in the case of speech development, because we have always the personal equation to consider and the condition of the infant at the particular time, but if we understood it better in terms of physiology, we might have more patience with the baby's efforts in learning to talk. We should certainly be less critical and less insistent on an immediate repetition

[1] Gifford, Mabel F., *Nervous and Mental Re-education.*

of difficult sounds or of words which the child cannot quite manage to say or to repeat.

When, to the infant, a single word stands for *an idea*, it is not so much that he is attempting to express a *thought*, as that he feels the need of *action* and of securing *attention*. His speech effort is socially motivated, and is an expression of his various activities or responses to environment. The quality of his efforts, the amount or degree of activity and effectiveness, are influenced by his physiological stage of development, by environment, and by the effort which the child must make to compel attention.

## Speech Learning    ,

We have said that the early speech habits of the child are " conditioned by environment ". The speed in speech development depends very much upon encouragement received in that environment—upon social urge, social pressure and competition for adult attention, as well as upon the physiological stage of development of the child.

A child may have had an adequate environment and sufficient social stimulation, and yet be slow in learning to talk. He may not talk at all until long after the period when children are usually able to express themselves. In such a case the parent becomes alarmed and seeks to find out the cause of the child's slowness in talking. A clinician, psychologist or speech therapist might suspect that one of the following conditions would be found in such a case. The child may be deaf, or some childhood illness may have slowed up his rate of development. There may be some slight remedial cause for the retardation, on the physical side, or the explanation may be that the mental development is retarded or even defective. If no abnormal condition is found on either the physical or the mental side, then we must look for the causes within the environment itself. Here we have to deal with the parents quite as much as with the child in order that they may aid in the elimination of the undesirable environmental factors which are retarding the child's speech progress. When a child hears well, is mentally normal, and there seems to be no physical or mental cause for retardation, then we usually find the cause within the home itself.

Most children not only babble considerably during the last half of the first year, but often have developed a considerable vocabulary of speech and even a few words, during the last few weeks of the first year. Other children show no such tendency, or at least develop no words until about the fifteenth to eighteenth month, and yet make rapid progress, once speech has really begun.[1]

We have already mentioned some causes for retardation in learning to talk. We have said that if there seems to be no degree of deafness present, no physical peculiarity and no mental deficiency, and yet the child does not learn to talk as early or as easily as have other children in the same family, we suspect some unfavourable psychic element to be the cause of the delay. We must look for the explanation within the child's customary environment, particularly in relation to the personalities and general social influences which surround the child.

Studies of infant growth and development have given us vocabulary norms for children at the ages of one, two and three years.[2] According to this study, children should possess an average of eight words at the end of the first year. The range found in the children studied by Waddle was from three to twenty-four words. Many parents believe that this number is too high an average, that it includes too small a number of children to be truly representative, and that only an exceptional child possesses a vocabulary of eight words at the end of the first year. So far as such objections have been registered, we have observed that the parents making these objections came from a different occupational level than those used by Waddle, as his " parents " belonged evidently to the professional group, or what Barr classified as the first occupational level, while the great majority of children

[1] Stern, Wm., *Psychology of Early Childhood*, Part II.
[2] Waddle, *Introd. to Child Psychology*, p. 166.

come from groups II to V, in Barr's classification.[1] Waddle's findings may be based on exceptional children, therefore, as his figures seem high, when compared with those obtained for other children.

The social differences in the child's environment may account for differences in the speed and acquisition of a serviceable vocabulary. Descoudres[2] has mentioned this in her study of children's vocabularies, in which she studied children representing families from a number of different occupational and social groups. In families where speech is encouraged, the stimulus to talk is stronger, and the setting more favourable to precocious speech development. She finds that speech develops earlier and more easily than in a less favourable setting.

It has been observed that children placed in foster homes in a new and better environment, frequently react surprisingly well to a more favourable opportunity, and that they reach in a short time a comparatively higher level of development than would have been possible had they remained in the original setting. They do not always reach the plane of the children of the foster parents, however.[3] Studies[4] of children in some of the state institutions for the blind, wherever such records are available, indicate that the blind child is slower in walking and talking than is the sighted child. Many blind children may develop speech which is greatly superior to that of the home environment however, when once they are placed in the school for the blind, where special educational advantages are given them.

### Significance of Environment

We suspect that if it were possible to check upon the home situation, we should find that those who do not progress at a rate which is within the range set by Waddle

---

[1] Woodworth, R., *Psychology*, "Barr's Occupational Classification," p. 48.

[2] Descoudres, A., *La Developpement*, 1923.

[3] Woodworth, *loc. cit.*, pp. 48–50.

[4] Burritt, O. H., *Reports of Pennsylvania Institution for the Blind.*

are less adequately socialized and less stimulated to talk by adults who surround them, than are children who show more language precocity.  That there are some dangers in precocious development is well known to clinicians and students of speech pathology, because they realize that it is all too easy to over-stimulate a precocious child, and to allow him to exhaust a great deal of nervous energy in the excitement of making early speech-responses under excessive adult pressure.  The writer has seen a number of such children whose parents and teachers have often guarded them against the strain of talking *too much*, as they may easily become fatigued and over-stimulated in the process.  One such child was a brilliant member of a nursery-school group, and at two-and-a-half she possessed a remarkable vocabulary, clear speech, and few if any letter substitutions or speech inaccuracies. Yet teachers and parents found it necessary to protect this child's active brain from literally wearing her out, in the tendency to talk incessantly to other children and adults.  She was still too young to be allowed to draw so unreservedly upon her strength as she was inclined to do.

Not only are we concerned with the appearance of speech at the normal time, but we find that we must sometimes guard a precocious child from *over-talking*. We need to protect such children from over-stimulation and exhaustion quite as much as we need to encourage the timid, delayed or retarded child to make the necessary efforts to speak.[1]

The reasons for speech delay or slowness in talking can only be discovered by adequate mental and physical examinations, or by careful study of the child's environment.  In the event of deafness, or in case it is suspected, a medical examination is necessary to test the hearing. If this is normal, we usually pass on to the mental examination given by a psychologist, in order that we may determine the child's mental age.  If by reason of retardation the child can take no tests involving language, a per-

MacCarthy, Dorothy, *Language and Speech Development*, 1930.

formance test may be given, such as the Pintner-Patterson Scale, which does not involve language responses.

If we find that none of these examinations has yielded positive evidence as to a physical cause, the retardation is felt to be due to environmental factors. The speech teacher must then find ways and means of stimulating the child to talk by means of little plays and games, using toys, pictures, objects of common use and the like. The speech worker needs special training in psychological principles and clinical practice in order to understand the child, to know when to modify her method, to observe when improvement is present, or when progress seems unduly slow. An examination by a psychiatrist or mental hygienist may yield fruitful results, and point out ways of dealing with the home situation. This is desirable to enable the worker to give the parents the necessary instructions for carrying on the work undertaken by the special teacher of speech. The special teacher who is to aid the child's speech development must have a broad, general foundation for her work, in order to deal successfully with the child, as a knowledge of the physiology and psychology of childhood is desirable to secure the fullest measure of co-operation from all concerned with the child's education. If one treats symptoms only, without removal of the cause, the speech may be temporarily improved, but the fundamentally disturbing factor may remain. To insist upon the child's coming up to an artistic standard of development, before he has learned to make himself intelligible, is putting the cart before the horse, and may intensify the already existing unfavourable condition, or even make the speech worse. This is especially true in many cases of stuttering. Any brilliant, over-talkative child may easily acquire the habit of stuttering. The stutterer needs not so much speech drill or speech exercises, as he needs sympathy and sufficient self-understanding to help him solve his difficulties, and to dispel any fears and anxieties concerning self-expression. Thus the aims and objectives of artistic

speech training and of corrective work are different—
a fact which is not generally recognized.

## Social Consequences of Wrong Speech Habits

Studies of child development show us that a " dwarfing "
or " short-circuiting " of the speech process may occur at
any one of a number of stages. It may be that the
environment is unfavourable, or that the child is physically
incapable of making the necessary effort to talk, if his
physiological development has not reached the proper
stage, or if he has been retarded by childhood illnesses.
If he is slow in gaining control of the larger fundamental
muscles involved in walking, he is usually slow in learning
to talk.[1]

Very few studies have been made to show the effect of
speech defects upon the unfolding of personality in the
child. Records of case histories given by various juvenile
court workers, clinicians, workers in speech pathology
and language development, show that the inculcation of
undesirable speech habits is unfavourable to the development of a personality free from timidity [2] and unhampered
by the feeling that something is out of focus in one's
relation to the world.[3]

Let us for a moment put aside the consideration of what
is happening to the infant who shows speech peculiarities
during the process of learning to talk, and consider what
may be the reaction of those about him. We have said
that savage tribes regard with suspicion any stranger to
their native tongue. Such a tribe might accept as normal
the speech and behaviour of a member of their own
tribe, even though his actions and the purport of his
words were most unusual, provided he speaks the
language which is the accepted mode of utterance in his
group.

[1] Blanton, S., *Child Guidance*, " Learning to Talk."
[2] Stinchfield, S. M., " Speech Defects as a Personnel Problem,"
*Jour. of Amer. Speech*, December 1926, pp. 148–52.
[3] Healy, W., *The Individual Delinquent*, pp. 220–23.

There is sometimes a striking similarity between the brilliant, erratic, flighty speech of a genius in his irresponsible moods, and that of the absolutely unbalanced person whom one sees in a clinic. The difference is in degree, quality and significance of the speech material used—its purpose, rather than in more obvious differences. Again, a feeble-minded or an insane person may speak with startling vividness and clearness of mental perception at times. Flight of ideas, word-salad speech and incoherent, disordered arrangement of words may alternate with perfectly lucid speech. In case of a developing psychosis, however, the lucid intervals tend to appear less and less frequently, and for shorter intervals during the onset of the mental disorder.[1]

Obviously, the speech of our own kind, or of our own group is what we expect to hear, and any deviation from accustomed speech strikes us at once as unusual, peculiar, even untrustworthy, so that we have a sort of mental reservation in the background of our consciousness, as to the value or reliability of the words uttered. If the speech sounds are different from those to which we are accustomed, we tend to concentrate upon how they sound, first of all, rather than upon the message which they are intended to convey. This corresponds to our mental attitude when we are listening to a foreign language. We must repeat to ourselves, first, sub-vocally, the word which has reached the auditory centre, and then the meaning begins to filter through to consciousness, if we are able to associate those sounds with previous experiences. The reaction time will necessarily be slower for new or unfamiliar speech than for speech which is at once perceived as familiar. Any speech peculiarity therefore tends to retard the reaction time in the listener, and to interfere with speed and clearness in forming a mental image of the words. Good speech is more economical, both for speaker and auditor, than is unusual, strange, or inaudible speech.

[1] White, Wm., *Outlines of Psychiatry*.

## *What is the Child's Native Tongue ?*

In speech as in dress and behaviour, we tend to be conservative. We prefer to hear accustomed sounds, whatever the cultural level represented. Language barriers are found to operate within a language as well as within geographically isolated areas, although such barriers differ in kind. While local differences will always exist, it might be useful in these days of international communication and speech if we could agree upon a common medium, for the purpose of international understanding— in a common English medium, for instance, as Mr. Henry Ford has suggested.[1] Suggestions regarding the development of a basic language are already current. Some countries possess an official and a colloquial language. If we should develop an international vocabulary, we might hope to reach some agreement as to what constitutes the most agreeable pronunciation, intonation, stress, accent, slang, and customary usage, even though we might prefer, at another time, to express ourselves in a simpler, more colloquial language. The true linguist is able to give the speech of different localities in the local mode of utterance, whatever the language he speaks. He may do this, even though his customary speech is distinctly representative of a different social group.

By " Native " speech we are accustomed to think of the local dialect of the community to which we belonged in childhood. We forget that speech is dynamic, changing from time to time, and even from day to day. It must do this in order to meet the demands of modern civilization. It changes to meet the economic needs of different social groups and of different nations. " Native " speech must be regarded as a living, vital force, developing endlessly with changes in custom, manners, social exigency, time and place. It must be " subject to change without notice ", because dictionaries can never anticipate the march of progress and must therefore always remain behind the mode, rather than up to the moment, as

---

[1] Ogden, C. K., *Debabelization*, 1931, p. 13.

B

language daily expands. What is current speech today, may become a vulgarism tomorrow. What is not accepted today, may be promoted to current usage in a week or a year if it fulfils certain needs and requirements better than do more familiar words. It is only by examining constantly the current speech habits of a social group whose taste in such things gives them an authoritative leadership, that we can know what constitutes desirable speech.

A good definition of normal speech is this : " Good speech is that which is inconspicuous, free from affectations of over- or under-articulation, and most readily accepted by the major group of cultured people whatever their geographical or social location." [1] It implies an orderly communication of thoughts in such a way as to require the least amount of effort to both speaker and hearer. Parents who represent good speech models themselves find it reflected in the speech of their children.

[1] MacLeod, E., *Lectures*, 1931.

# CHAPTER II

## THE SPEECH OF CHILDHOOD: SPEECH DEFECTS CLASSIFIED

### NORMAL AND ABNORMAL SPEECH IN EARLY CHILDHOOD

#### Speech Patterns

WE have given some time to the discussion of speech development in infancy, and have traced some of the causes of speech difficulties to their origin in childhood. We now wish to consider the speech characteristics of early childhood, as the child passes beyond the early speech-experimental stage, and to ascertain if possible, some of the consequences of unfavourable speech-development upon adult life and personality.

Most writers agree that at about the time the child learns to walk he often becomes so engrossed in the process of locomotion at the end of the first year that he seems to require all of his energy for this important achievement. His acquisition of new sounds often slows up for a few weeks, until he has mastered the new " skill ", after which he returns usually with renewed energy to the word-acquisition habit. Locomotion only *seems* to retard the speech development, for as a matter of fact, the new experiences gained in walking, new understanding of objects and things in terms of a third dimension have enabled the child to discover a new world for himself. Size, shape, distance, contours of objects and inter-relationships have invested them with new and unsuspected qualities. He now begins to gain what the Germans call " configurations " or images which group themselves about other experiences and serve as a focal point for the acquisition of new knowledge.

Just as in colour-vision, where every patch of colour

is influenced by every other patch in its environment, so we feel that in speech, the configurations which a child gains of speech-motor activities are not entirely due to auditory patterns. The child often looks observantly at the lips of a speaker, or endeavours through a study of facial expression to grasp meanings more completely, and will make a fresh start in the attempt to imitate the sound heard. A two-year-old may often be broken of a letter substitution by merely showing him, calmly and casually as a sort of play or game, how the adult makes these sounds. If the child is not a stutterer, and the adult does not scold or " nag ", a few repetitions of this act will often suffice to give the child the eye-motor imagery necessary to produce the sound correctly. With an observant child who easily learns by the visual process, new habits are formed very quickly in this way. With a feeble-minded, retarded or backward child, sometimes no amount of observation seems to enable him to make much improvement, as he is not eye-minded, but depends almost entirely upon auditory stimuli for making speech sounds. Undoubtedly most of us depend chiefly upon auditory impressions for our stimuli in learning to talk, but this does not preclude the possibility of employing visual methods as well, when we find that it is a short-cut to the correction of speech inaccuracies. The sooner such an " inaccuracy " is removed, the better for the child. Sometimes a child will imitate motor movements and the *look* of the letters or sounds better than he can possibly reproduce the sounds by ear, especially if he happens to be one in whom visual and motor images predominate over auditory ones. The visuo-motor image is not so necessary and may be of little or no importance to the child who learns readily by ear.

Speech pathologists find that with dull, backward or mentally deficient children, and even with some of very low grades of intelligence, the visual method is a very useful addition to the auditory. In one of the classes for retarded children in the London Schools the writer saw the teacher gaining excellent results with these children when she merely went through the action of articulating certain sounds silently and then told the children to give verbally the sound she was illustrating. After a little drill, the eye-motor stimulus was sufficient to stimulate each child to give the desired sounds correctly, when such sounds were simple ones which could be made with lips or front of tongue, such as *oo, ee, ah, p, b, t, d, th,* and sometimes *l.*[1]

## The Question of Imagery

It is impossible for one to know, in the earlier years, whether the child is primarily audito-motor, visuo-motor, tactuo-motor or tactuo-audile, and to determine just what combination of sensory discrimination and motor reaction - tendencies predominates. The psychologist claims that the child does not usually isolate one factor out of a total sensory experience, and attend exclusively to it, be it vision, sound or touch. We are finding that the configuration or conception which a child has of any sensory experience, depends largely upon the way in which a given sensory experience is compounded or upon innate tendencies in the child. If the child tends to be more attentive to visual stimuli, he may also at the same time be attending to other components in the situation, such as touch, size, shape, smoothness or roughness. It may be that gustatory or olfactory impressions enter vividly into the experience. The same stimulus given to two children at the same time, and under identical controlled conditions, might mean different things to each. The same experience, if presented to the same child at some other time, might be interpreted quite differently than when it was originally presented.

This seems to us to be significant in understanding the learning processes involved in speech, because we might save much time and energy in cases where a speech difficulty appears in early childhood, if we could present the sound which we wish the child to imitate, in such a

[1] Tollett St., *Special Class in Speech,* 1931.

way as to favour its perception by the child as a desirable thing to imitate. Parents might endeavour through simple plays, games and experiences of a suitable level, to stimulate the child's understanding and to enrich the scope of his experiences in fields in which he may be responsive. In this way little defects might be eliminated without ever being called directly to the child's attention, and without remaining in his consciousness long enough to become set or habitual.[1]

If we wait until the linkage between seeing, hearing, and making the various speech sounds is well set, firmly rooted, and habitual, it is not only more difficult to eradicate permanently, but it is much more unlikely that we shall be able to overcome the faulty speech habits. The child cannot acquire the new sound as perfectly as might have been the case had he been corrected at the outset.[2]

Even though a child may outgrow a minor speech difficulty, by exercise of his own powers of observation and imitation, he usually can do so much quicker under unobtrusive skilled advice. This may be given by parents working in co-operation with the special teacher. Many speech disorders apparent in childhood are also found at a later period. Some of them may appear for the first time in early childhood, or in later childhood, or in adolescence, but the majority of speech disturbances of the remedial type appear in childhood. Some are outgrown in the case of observant, intelligent children, or those with good auditory imagery. Many yield easily to the follow-up work done by parents, after a few special lessons with a skilled teacher. That this is so, is evident from the many letters which have been received by the lecturer on speech disorders for the British Broadcasting Corporation, which were at the disposal of the writer.[3] Many types of difficulties persisting into later childhood

[1] *Psychologies of* 1930, " Configurational Psychologies," Köhler, p. 143 ; Koffka, p. 161.

[2] Koffka, K., *The Growth of Mind*, " The Mind of the New-born Babe."

[3] MacLeod, Eileen, *The Child's Speech*, Radio Talks, 1930–31.

have been cleared up with a little special advice, given over the radio, or in some cases by letter, or by personal conferences.[1] Parents should be on guard, however, against the commonly expressed opinion that children will " outgrow " defects in speech.

That many parents are able to profit from simple instructions regarding the speech-learning process, and to apply them successfully to the training of their children, is evident from the number of letters received by Eileen MacLeod, lecturer on speech disorders with the British Broadcasting Corporation. Following a series of simple talks to parents, the speaker received letters from all parts of the Empire, describing some of the speech difficulties of children in various homes, such letters asking for advice, or seeking interviews. Certain types of articulatory defects in normal children, described to the parents in detail, were dealt with by Miss MacLeod at King's College Hospital Speech Clinic, and her correspondence shows that some of the mothers were able to remove the difficulties by learning how to deal with them at home. These children might not have " outgrown " it by themselves, but by receiving some unobtrusive help, through the mother's special training, they were able to make rapid progress in acquiring better speech habits.

In the beginning stages of stuttering it is true that if a parent pays very little attention to the difficulty, so far as directing the child's attention to the disorder is concerned, the tendency to stumble and to speak incoherently will disappear with a little casual and sympathetic aid on the part of the parent. A younger child in the effort to keep pace with an older one, often stumbles stammers or stutters in trying to get the words out too hastily. It is unwise to set the habit in the child's consciousness, but parents may repeat in an entirely normal

[1] MacLeod, Eileen, *The Child's Speech, Radio Talks*, 1930-1931.

NOTE. — The references to Gestalt Psychology refer primarily to experiments now being carried on at the Psychological Institute, University of Berlin, under direction of Professor Köhler, the results of which have not yet been published.

fashion the sentences or phrases which the child has found difficult. Often a child will immediately repeat a sentence correctly after having heard it once.

It is very unwise to scold a child for faults of speech, or to be insistent upon his repeating words. It is still worse to make him repeat isolated letter-sounds. No one begins to talk by rehearsing consonants repeatedly! Calmness, quietness, good speech as an example and freedom from undue haste or excitement are the best ways to help a small child to talk naturally. The baby's speech, we have said, is more easily acquired and more natural than the speech of an adult who is making an attempt to acquire a new language. We should foster natural ease in language acquisition and not make the child unduly self-conscious in the process.

The majority of forms of speech disorders have already been extensively treated by various authors. Definitions of the familiar types have been given elsewhere, and we shall consider here only those forms which we believe to be of special interest to parents, teachers of speech and clinicians, in the process of treating disorders of speech, or in their prevention.

Before we can proceed further with definitions and descriptions of common disorders of speech in children or adults, it is necessary to set boundaries by offering a practical classification of the more familiar deviations from normal speech. We offer for guidance in reading the next few chapters, the classification recommended by the American Society for the Study of Disorders of Speech, as a result of its studies following the publication of its *Dictionary of Terms* dealing with disorders of speech.[1]

### CLASSIFICATION OF DISORDERS OF SPEECH

#### I. DYSARTHRIA (See Chapter V)

Defects of articulation due to lesions of the nervous system :

*A*. ANARTHRIA—INARTICULATENESS.

*B*. BRADYARTHRIA—LABOURED SPEECH.

*C*. MOGIARTHRIA—ATAXIC SPEECH.

---

[1] Robbins-Stinchfield, 1931.

## II. DYSLALIA

(*a*) lalling.
(*b*) oral inaccuracy.
(*c*) phonetic defects.

Functional and organic defects of articulation :

*A*. ALALIA—MUTISM.

    *a*. alalia cophotica—deaf-mutism.
    *b*. alalia organica.
    *c*. alalia physiologica—physiologic mutism.
    *d*. alalia prolongata—delayed speech.

        1. auditory dumbness.
        2. hearing mutism.
        3. mutitas prolongata.

*B*. BARBARALALIA—FOREIGN DIALECT. (*Note.*—Foreign accent comes under dysrhythmia.)

    *a*. provincialism.

*C*. BARYLALIA—CLUTTERING.

*D*. IDIOLALIA—INVENTED LANGUAGE.

    *a*. idioglossia.
    *b*. pathological language.

*E*. PARALALIA—Lisping—Sound substitution.

*F*. PEDOLALIA—INFANTILE PERSEVERATION.

*G*. RHINOLALIA—nasal, inarticulate speech.

    *a*. rhinolalia megauvulica, due to elongation of uvula.
    *b*. rhinolalia microuranica, due to insufficient length of soft palate.
    *c*. rhinolalia uranoschismatica—cleft-palate speech.
    *d*. rhinolalia uranotraumatica, due to palatal injury.

## III. DYSLOGIA

Difficulty in the expression of ideas by speech, due to psychoses :

*A*. AGRAMMALOGIA—INCOHERENT SPEECH.

*B*. ALOGIA—ABSENCE OF IDEAS.

    *a*. alogia idiotica—idiotic mutism.

*C*. BRADYLOGIA—SLUGGISH SPEECH.

    *a*. bradyphrasia.

*D*. CATALOGIA—VERBIGERATION.

    *a*. perseveration.

        1. echolalia—echoic speech.
        2. stereotypy.

*E*. Paralogia—Irrelevant Speech.
*F*. Polylogia—Excessive Loquacity.
   *a*. logorrhea (speech pressure).
   *b*. polyphrasia (blustering, punning, rhyming speech).
   *c*. hyperphrasia.
*G*. Tachylogia—morbid rapidity of speech : Agitologia.
   *a*. tachyphrasia.

### IV. DYSPHASIA (See Re-Classification, Chapter VII)

Impairment of language, due to weakened mental imagery : through disease, shock or injury.

*A*. Motor Aphasia.
   *a*. Agraphia.
   *b*. Amusia.
   *c*. Amimia.
   *d*. Logaphasia—Articulatory Aphasia.
      1. aphemia.
      2. articulatory word amnesia.
      3. mental dumbness.
      4. motor vocal aphasia.
      5. psychic dumbness.
   *e*. Motor Alexia.

*B*. Sensory Aphasia.
   *a*. Auditory Aphasia.
      1. mind-deafness.
         sensory amusia (*a*. tone-deafness).
         logokyphosis—word-deafness.
      2. psychic deafness.
   *b*. Visual Aphasia.
      1. intellectual blindness.
      2. mental blindness.
      3. psychic blindness.
         *a*. agnosia.
         *b*. alexia—word-blindness.[1]

*C*. Mixed Aphasia.
   *a*. Agrammaphasia—Syntactical Aphasia—Word - salad Speech.
   *b*. Aphasia—Speechlessness.
   *c*. Bradyphasia—Groping Speech.
   *d*. Cataphasia—Repetitious Speech.
   *e*. Paraphasia—Word Substitution.

*D*. Total Aphasia.
   *a*. aphasia universalis.

---

[2] Ref., *Dyslexia*, p. 32.

## V. DYSPHEMIA

Variable disorders of speech due to psychoneuroses :

*A*. AGITOPHEMIA—nervous, agitated speech.

*B*. APHEMIA—DUMBNESS.

    *a*. aphemia hysterica—hysterical mutism.
    *b*. aphemia pathematica—due to fright or passion (lalophobia).
    *c*. aphemia plastica—voluntary muteness.
    *d*. aphemia spasmodica—spasmodic dumbness.

*C*. PARAPHEMIA—NEUROTIC LISPING.

*D*. SPASMOPHEMIA—STAMMERING—STUTTERING.

| | |
|---|---|
| *a*. aphonia spastica. | *i*. logospasm. |
| *b*. broken rhythm. | *j*. mogilalia. |
| *c*. cluttering. | *k*. molilalia. |
| *d*. convulsive hesitation. | *l*. spasmodic speech. |
| *e*. dysarthria. | *m*. spastic aphonia. |
| *f*. dysphemia. | *n*. speech blocking. |
| *g*. dysphonia spastica. | *o*. speech hesitation. |
| *h*. linguæ hesitantia. | *p*. speech stumbling. |

    1. spasmophemia clonica—stuttering.
    2. spasmophemia cryptica—silent stammering.
    3. spasmophemia tonica—stammering.
        *a*. dysarthria literalis.

## VI. DYSPHONIA

Defects of voice : This includes all disorders of phonation due to organic or functional disorders of vocal cords, or to defective respiration.

*A*. APHONIA—absence of voice.

    *a*. aphonia apophatica, due to negativism (also a dyslogia or a dysphemia).
    *b*. aphonia hysterica—hysterical aphonia (also a dysphemia).
    *c*. aphonia organica—due to structural anomalies of the larynx.
    *d*. aphonia paralytica (also a dysarthria).
    *e*. aphonia paranoica (also a dyslogia).
    *f*. aphonia pathematica, due to fright, or passion (also a dyslogia or a dysphemia).
        1. phonophobia.
    *g*. aphonia spastica—spastic aphonia (also a dysphemia).
    *h*. aphonia traumatica—due to injury to the larynx.

*B*. BARYPHONIA—THICK VOICE.
    *a*. dull voice.

*C*. GUTTUROPHONIA—GUTTURAL VOICE.
    *a*. throaty voice.

*D*. Hypophonia—Whispered Voice.

   *a*. voluntary whispering.

*E*. Idiophonia : individual characteristics of voice :

| | | |
|---|---|---|
| *a*. acute voice. | *i*. infantile. | *q*. sepulchral. |
| *b*. coarse. | *j*. lour. | *r*. shrill. |
| *c*. flat. | *k*. monotonous. | *s*. sombre. |
| *d*. gloomy. | *l*. muffled. | *t*. strident. |
| *e*. grave. | *m*. passive. | *u*. subdued. |
| *f*. growling. | *n*. rasping. | *v*. toneless. |
| *g*. hard. | *o*. raucous. | *w*. whining. |
| *h*. harsh. | *p*. rough. | |

*F*. Megaphonia—Morbidly Loud Voice.

*G*. Metallophonia—Metallic Voice.

   *a*. grating voice.

*H*. Microphonia—Weak Voice.

*I*. Paraphonia—morbid alterations of voice.

   *a*. paraphonia adenopathica, due to certain glandular diseases.
   *b*. paraphonia amazonica—virago speech (in women).
   *c*. paraphonia athymica, change of voice in depression.
   *d*. paraphonia copiaca, change of voice in fatigue.
   *e*. paraphonia eunuchoidia, falsetto quality of voice in eunuchs.
   *f*. paraphonia geratica, high, cracked voice of old age.
   *g*. paraphonia microischica, change of voice in lowered vitality.
   *h*. paraphonia neurasthenica—neurasthenic voice.
   *i*. paraphonia pubetica—harsh, irregular, breaking voice of puberty.

      1. dysphonia puberum.

*J*. Pneumaphonia—Breathy Voice.

   *a*. aspirate voice.

*K*. Rhinophonia—Nasal Voice.

   *a*. nasality.  *b*. nasalizing.  *c*. rhinism.  *d*. rhinolalia clausa.

*L*. Tanyphonia—Thin Voice.

   *a*. pinched voice.

*M*. Trachyphonia—Hoarseness.

   *a*. trachyphonia ecclesiastica, due to clergyman's sore throat.
   *b*. trachyphonia infiltrata, due to infiltration from diseased tonsils, adenoids, sinuses, etc.

*N*. Tromophonia—Tremulous Voice.

## VII. DYSRHYTHMIA

Defects of rhythm (other than stuttering) :

*A*. DYSRHYTHMIA  PNEUMAPHRASIA — DEFECTS  OF  BREATH GROUPING.

*B*. DYSRHYTHMIA PROSODIA—DEFECTS OF STRESS PLACEMENT.

*C*. DYSRHYTHMIA TONIA—DEFECTS OF INFLECTION.

Terms recommended for common use are given in the larger type. The preferred scientific term is given, together with its more commonly used equivalent or synonym, when one is recommended. Less important or less frequently used terms are in the smaller case type. Some cross-classification occurs, as a number of disorders may occur in several different diseases, or under several different headings. The attempt is made in this arrangement to give the student an outline of practically all of the commonly found disorders of speech, such as appear in home, school and speech clinic, and to so group them that they may come under one of seven main headings, *i.e.*, dysarthria, dyslalia, dyslogia, dysphasia, dysphemia, dysphonia or dysrhythmia. These terms have been worked out in order that speech disorders might be identified, using the descriptive *prefix* " dys ", and a causal *suffix*. In order to systematize the classification, it was necessary for the committee on terminology to coin a number of new terms having old prefixes, frequently defining the older and better-known terms as synonymous with the coined ones. Thus POLYPHRASIA, a form of dyslogia, is defined as synonymous with the newly coined term POLYLOGIA, having an ending which at once shows it to be a dyslogia. As the definitions and pronunciation have been given elsewhere, we shall not include them with our classification here, and the reader is referred to the *Dictionary of Terms* for such information, if desired.

# CHAPTER III

## COMMON SPEECH DIFFICULTIES OF CHILDHOOD :
## DYSLEXIA AND DYSLALIA

### Dyslexia : in the non-Reader Child

IF a child is unable to profit by reading instruction in the first grade, and comes to the end of the first or second year with little or no improvement in reading, it retards his progress so seriously as to place him in the position of the very backward child. Even though he begins to read slowly in the second year, he is often greatly retarded because of the early delay in learning to read. He is also liable to make errors in writing, to misspell, mispronounce, misread and stumble even after he has mastered the elementary reading process sufficiently to do oral reading. Here it would seem that the most profitable method, educationally, would be to find out in which of the sensory realms the child is most responsive, and then to attempt to build up associations between the weaker types of imagery and those which are more vivid in his case.[1]

Suppose a child has been referred because she not only has careless, mumbled speech, but she also mispronounces, misspells and writes incoherently. We find on examination that she tends to respond very well to visual stimuli, but that her auditory impressions are hazy and inaccurate. It would be a waste of time if we continued to try to train her primarily through the auditory method in such a case, whereas if we utilize the well-functioning visual imagery, through the " look-and-say " method, she will become more observant of fundamental differences between words, and we may later link

---

[1] Stinchfield, S. M., *Speech Pathology*, 1928, pp. 1–22.

her visual observation with more adequate auditory impressions than she has hitherto been able to acquire. We should do the child an injustice and expect too much of her were we to assume that with a little training we could cause the " amnesia " to disappear.  She will always be a better visual type than an auditory, but we may strengthen by training, the bonds or linkages between her inherent capacities and those in which she is weak.[1]

In the treatment of stuttering and lalling the theory has been advanced that such inadequate speech is due to transient auditory or visual amnesia, and that by strengthening the visual impressions, primarily, one might eradicate the speech defect.  We feel that imagery is a matter of innate endowment, and that we are following a better method if we examine first the child's mental processes so as to find out, if possible, whether he is specially limited in visual, auditory or kinæsthetic imagery. Then the most economical method is to employ the images of the type to which he best responds, and to utilize them so far as possible in building up clear images of the words, sounds, pictures or phrases or sentences which he can easily retain or utilize : and after having done this, to progress to the strengthening of the bonds between the clear images he has, and those in which he is deficient.  We believe that his " amnesia ", if we can call it such, is not a transient thing, but relatively fixed and permanent, and only subject to change after careful investigation and re-education.  Differences in innate capacities and endowment account for many of the differences in clearness of perception and imagery.

Mary B. was a child of ten years of age referred to a child guidance clinic.  She stumbled a great deal in reading and misspelled many words in school.  She had great difficulty in reading aloud.  It was found that her hearing was normal, and she imitated sounds on various pitches, without difficulty.  In writing, however, she tended to spell phonetically.  She was not trained to

[1] Dearborn, Lord, Carmichael, *Special Disabilities in Learning to Read and Write*, Harvard Monog. in Educa., 1925.

look at words, or to recognize letter-sequences. It was felt that she needed eye-speech training and improvement in visual impressions. After a little practice on auditory images, through which she became encouraged by her successes, it was not difficult to make the transition to the look-and-say method and to secure improvement in a short training period of several lessons.

## DYSLEXIA [1]

The following classification of disabilities in reading which are closely associated with speech defects, is recommended by the Nomenclature Committee of the American Society for the Study of Disorders of Speech. The detailed outline has been prepared in collaboration with Dr. Thomas H. Eames of the Harvard University Psycho-Educational Clinic. As the entire classification will shortly be published elsewhere, we shall confine ourselves to an abbreviated form for practical use in the speech clinic.

As teachers of speech correction are often required to give remedial reading and speech treatment in the public schools and in many of the child guidance clinics, it has been found necessary to extend the classification of speech disorders, mentioned in Chapter II, so as to include some suggestions for the speech worker who deals with various forms of reading disability and associated speech disorders. It is important to refer such cases to a competent optometrist for special examination and recommendations, and for the speech worker to deal with such cases under medical direction. She needs also to be skilled in the application of the recent methods for dealing with the non-reader child, such as the Fernald Method in use in the Psychological Clinic of the University of California at Los Angeles, or of the Monroe Method, in use in the Chicago Institute for Juvenile Research. The

[1] Nomenclature Committee, American Society for the Study of Disorders of Speech. S. D. Robbins, chairman, Boston (unpublished revision).

Gates Educational Material in use at Columbia University is also recommended, as well as methods described by Gray, University of Chicago, Stone, *Oral and Silent Reading*, Daniel Starch in *Educational Measurements*, Orton and Travis, State University of Iowa.

## CLASSIFICATION OF DYSLEXIA

*A*. ALEXIA—Complete inability to read anything.
1. Pathological, due to an actual lesion.
2. Psychological.
   *a*. ANORTHOGRAPHIA—spelling disability due to conditions imposed upon the child to which he cannot adjust.

*B*. BARYLEXIA—Careless in reading with marked elision and assimilation as in speech defect known as " cluttering ".

*C*. BRADYLEXIA—Slow recognition of words, a stage or degree of Psychological Alexia.

*D*. CATALEXIA—Re-reading, repetition.

*E*. PALINLEXIA—Reading backward.

*F*. PARALEXIA—Constant or intermittent letter substitutions.
1. paralexia anatropica—inversions ($A$ for$V$).
2. paralexia antitropica—reversals ($b$ for $d$).
3. paralexia metathetica—transpositions ($ad$ for $da$).
4. paralexia homeomorphica—substitution of letters having similar forms ($f$ for $t$).
5. paralexia tychotropica—random letter substitution ($l$ for $p$).

## CAUSES OF DYSLEXIA

1. Agnotica, due to unknown or uncertain causes.
2. Amphidexotica, due to ambidexterity and the resulting lack of unilateral cerebral dominance.
3. Anopsica, due to total blindness.
4. Aphasica, due to impaired mental imagery in aphasia or dysphasia.
5. Brachymnesica, due to apparent or initial lowered memory function.

   *a*. Brachymnesica acoustica, due to lowered auditory function.
   *b*. Brachymnesica optica, due to lowered visual function.
6. Cophotica, due to defective hearing.
7. Dysopsia, due to defective vision.
8. Dysstereoptica, due to deficiencies of fusion.

C

9. Idiotica, due to mental deficiency.
10. Emotio-pathematica, due to emotionalism.
11. Pathologica, due to a lesion which is usually found in the left supramarginal and angular gyri.

Among the chief causes of defective vision the following are of special importance in dealing with the non-reader child.

*A*. Hypermetropia or far-sightedness.
*B*. Myopia or near-sightedness.
*C*. Astigmia or astigmatism.
*D*. Heterophoria or tendency of visual lines to deviate from parallelism.
*E*. Heterotropia—actual deviation of visual lines from parallelism.
*F*. Amblyopia—dimness of vision without organic lesion of the eye.
*G*. Scotoma—a blind area in the retina.
*H*. Anopsia—total blindness.

Deficiencies in fusion are primarily due to the following :—

*A*. Anorthopia or distorted vision.
*B*. Heterophoria.  (See *D* above.)
*C*. Heterotropia.  (See *E* above.)
*D*. Amblyopia (unilateral).  (See *F* above.)
*E*. Monoptopathia—neural lesions affecting one eye or its neural connections.

### Dyslalia

Dyslalia is discussed here, because it is one of the speech disorders which is most frequently found in childhood, whereas dysarthria is more commonly found in adulthood, since it is most frequently found to be due to lesions of the central nervous system, which are less frequently found in children than in adults. We have deferred the discussion of dysarthria to a later chapter.

Theories have been advanced from time to time in regard to the occurrence of defective imagery in speech-defective children. Swift and Bluemel have written favouring the transient visual and auditory amnesia theories. Orton offers evidence of the inheritability of certain defects such as word-blindness, word-deafness, handedness and other limitations which appear in the speech clinic and in the child-guidance clinics. Frequently the possession of a mild or serious speech defect is the reason for referring the child to the speech clinic, even though it is properly an educational problem of quite another type, demanding special remedial measures in reading, quite apart from speech rehabilitation.

The frequency with which such children are referred to speech clinics requires a few words of explanation. Many of them are found to be retarded one or more years in grade, although possessing average intelligence. They are simply unable to profit by the usual instruction in reading, and even by the end of the first year in school may still be unable to pass the simplest reading tests for that grade. The frequency of the appearance of the non-reader child, sometimes called an "aphasic", has been commented upon much of late in the speech-correction literature of America, England, Germany and Austria.

Lalling, oral inactivity and phonetic defects are common in such children, along with the special handicaps of dyslexia and agnosia, visual, auditory, or ideational difficulties.

### ALALIA or MUTISM

#### (A. Organic; B. Functional Absence of Speech)

##### Organic Alalia

This form of mutism may be due to malformation or imperfect innervation of the tongue and other organs of speech or hearing, or to lesions within the brain and other parts of the central nervous system affecting the speech function. We find that such mutism may range all the way from the obstinate, voluntary silence of the psychotic and hysterical child or adult to deaf-mutism, mental deficiency and idiocy.

The normal child has a good many sounds and sometimes a few words at the end of the first year.[1] When a child shows no signs of talking by the fifteenth to eighteenth month, it is well to delay a little longer perhaps before feeling unduly alarmed.[2] Many boys begin to talk later

---

[1] Fenton, J., *The Psychology of Babyhood.*
[2] Blanton, S. and M., *Child Guidance.*

than girls, but they have usually quite a number of words by the end of the eighteenth month. A physical examination is advisable when a child shows no tendency to talk until long after the age when other children of the same family began to talk, and when he seems to show no signs of developing overt speech. Contrary to the common notion, lack of speech is rarely due to " tongue-tie ", or to any defect in the speech organs themselves. Alalia may be of the organic type, when the tongue or any of the organs of speech or hearing, or the brain cells are defective. We speak of it as functional when hysterical or voluntary muteness occurs. The term *Aphemia* is often used to cover this type of speech disorder. Complete dumbness is found in a number of the psychoneuroses, silence for varying periods of time alternating with extremely loquacious moods, as in the case of manic-depressive insanity or in dementia præcox. It has also been called a form of articulatory aphasia, the organs of speech and power of innervation remaining, but the muteness being of central origin, and presumably under voluntary control, in the psychoneuroses and hysterias. The patient *can* talk, but *won't* talk in such cases.


## DEAF-MUTISM (Organic)

Let us consider forms of deafness which occur early in the life of the child, and before speech has developed. We do not wish to take a biased attitude of emotionality, nor one which is influenced solely by the spirit of scientific interest. The deaf child has already enough difficulty, without being further discriminated against, and we know that he is usually able to earn his own living and to take his place in normal community life, whenever his handicap is not unduly great. Although the problem of the deaf child is not so serious as that of the blind child, it is true that unless the fact of deafness is ascertained early in the child's development, every month of delay may make it increasingly difficult for him to make a normal social adjustment. Failure to develop speech interferes with a child's ability to make normal social contacts, and the older he grows before remedial measures are taken, the more difficult it becomes for him to make up for lost time, educationally. He may even remain permanently " retarded by deprivation ".

Many books have been written on the subject of deafness and the problems of the deaf, and we shall not concern ourselves here with these, except as they relate to the problem of speech-retardation in the deaf child. Even though the degree of deafness may be improved by remedial measures, there usually exists a speech impediment in the case of the child who is born deaf, or who is deprived of hearing before he has learned to talk. The child lacks the auditory discrimination which hearing gives to the average person, and without auditory cues, he is unable to know when he is speaking correctly or intelligibly. Even in cases of " total " deafness, speech may be developed by corrective measures. The physical handicap of deafness itself is a sufficient burden to the child so afflicted, without his speech remaining inarticulate and unintelligible. Unless the deaf child is trained through the remaining sensory avenues, he tends to develop only a few primitive sounds, or else no speech at all.

The classification of deafness usually given is that summarized by Best [1] : (a) congenital, hereditary deafness, (b) adventitious deafness, (c) infantile or sporadic deafness due to diseases, (d) miscellaneous forms of deafness. It rarely results from blows, but appears frequently in adult life, particularly in old age, from a hardening of the middle ear structures, as a result of arterial sclerosis.

### Prevention of Deafness

The elimination of all causes of deafness is as yet largely an ideal, although there has been a great advance as a result of improved hygiene, early medical attention, and prevention of unfortunate consequences from childhood diseases. This handicap has not as yet been pre-

[1] Best, H., *The Deaf*, 1914.

vented in infancy to the same extent as blindness.[1] It is therefore probable that deaf children will continue to be referred to the speech clinics for some years to come, and that the teacher of speech should be prepared to undertake the training of the partially or " *totally* " deaf child.[2]

We believe that many cases of lisping or of indistinct utterance on *s* and *z* sounds are due to the fact that there is in such cases a high-frequency deafness, and that the child or adult does not hear the high-pitched *s* sound accurately, and therefore cannot give it correctly. It is possible that we now and again confuse such cases of high-frequency deafness with what we assume to be poor auditory imagery. Teachers of speech often express surprise at the persistence of a near-lisp, even after a student has apparently eliminated it. The fact may be that the student is unaware of the return of the lisp, after it has been corrected, due to the fact that the ear is defective for certain pitches. The student can make a mechanical correction for the time being, but is unable to carry it over permanently, without long and tedious drill. It is quite possible that he may never be able to eliminate his speech inaccuracy. We believe that such cases occur.

## Education of the Deaf Child

The modern deaf child or adult is far less affected by the affliction of inadequate hearing than was the case a few generations ago. Special educational methods, lip-reading, the sign-language, vocational guidance and instruction in practically all the common school subjects have given him the necessary tools with which to cope with his difficulty. If he is capable of being trained in lip-reading, there is no occasion for him to learn the

[1] Best, H., *The Deaf*, p. 309.

[2] NOTE.—The italics are the writer's own. What we call "total deafness" is sometimes found to be only partial. There may be tonal gaps or islands of deafness, and yet parts of the tonal scale which the child hears and understands quite well. The question of *total deafness* is still a controversial one.

manual alphabet. If his deafness has been complicated by other handicaps such as retardation, mental or physical, he may not be able to acquire the skill necessary to read the lips and may be forced to depend wholly upon the sign language. Artificial aids to hearing and improved knowledge of the physiology of the ear have placed the deaf person in a more favourable economic position today than formerly.

## Personality of the Deaf Child

Because of the nature of deafness, it is true that the deaf child seems to be less sociable than the blind child. Socialization of the deaf child at an early age is a very important matter. If the child feels too keenly the extent of his affliction, because of attitude of parents or of other children, his personality may become considerably warped before he is old enough to go to school, or to attend special classes. Helen Keller [1] has described in detail the mental suffering of the deaf-blind child in a world where nobody seems to understand. She describes typical " temper-tantrums " in which she frequently indulged, before the coming of her teacher, Miss Sullivan. Her entire horizon and outlook on life was broadened and enormously modified by the new and absorbing miracle of communication.

Formerly the education of the deaf child was most often undertaken in a State school or special institution. Recently special classes for the deaf child have been offered in many public schools, and many parents prefer this type of education, as the child attends day school, but remains with his family at other times, and is assured of more normal family life. The child also learns very early to adjust to life as he finds it, and as he must meet it, sooner or later, independently.[2]

The teaching of speech to the totally deaf child is a highly specialized form of work, requiring special training. The teacher in speech correction should have a knowledge

[1] Keller, H., *The World I Live In*.
Keller, H., *The Story of My Life*.
[2] Best, H., *The Deaf*, pp. 309–324.

of the special methods employed in teaching the deaf child, and should know something about the psychological problems associated with deafness. She should be well-grounded in phonetics, lip-reading, physical education [1] and speech science generally, as applied to the speech-education of the deaf child.

It is the practice in most of the eastern women's colleges of the United States to require a deaf girl to take preliminary training in some good school of lip-reading before she enters college. The instructors in speech correction in the colleges find it a great advantage to have the girl follow up her lip-reading for a part of the time while she is in college, in order not to lose the skill she has already acquired. Deafness is bound to enter into the question of vocational choice on leaving college, and the greater the assurance and belief in her speech understanding, the better are the girl's chances for making a satisfactory adjustment and finding normal happiness in life situations.

In the case of the congenitally deaf child, the problem is more acute than is the case where deafness is acquired, unless this deafness has come about as the result of one of the childhood diseases occurring before the child has learned to talk. In the latter case the plight of the deaf child is practically identical with that of the child born deaf. In order to compete successfully with other children or with adults in the home situation, the deaf child must be trained to use whatever remnant of hearing remains, and to utilize remaining sensory avenues such as the kinæsthetic and visual, especially, more expertly than does the non-handicapped child. For the child of normal intelligence the lip-reading method is preferred. Children pick this up very quickly. Adults who make slow progress

---

[1] NOTE.—Deaf children are rather prone to respiratory diseases. Exercises to develop the lung capacity and to improve oral and nasal hygiene are important. Rhythm, through kinæsthetic sensation, may supply some of the deficiencies due to lack of hearing, and where there is a remnant of hearing, the amplifier and loud speaker have made it possible for some children to hear the sound of the human voice for the first time (Clarke School for the Deaf, Northampton, Mass.).

in lip-reading are generally those who refuse to accept the fact of deafness, and who show a perverse mental attitude, stubbornness, pride and fear of humiliation. Because of their deafness they are apt to become unduly suspicious about any sounds or words which they do not understand. Such an attitude in either child or adult is most unfavourable to rapid progress in learning to read the lips, and in adjusting to one's handicap. The unfavourable mental attitude often strengthens with long continued deafness, and renders the person disagreeable, unpopular, and disliked by friends and relatives who must continually deal with him.[1]

Even though a child is not totally deaf, the nervous strain incident to trying to *hear* is reduced by training the eyes to *see* what is said. Education of the deaf promotes their mental, physical and moral welfare, often enabling them to compete successfully in difficult fields. Whatever the educator may do to prevent the isolation, pathos and unsocial development of the deaf child or adult, is a step in the right direction.

One may minimize a handicap by paying no obvious or conspicuous attention to it. One may develop interest in and patience towards deaf children and aid them in normal development by making them feel that they are in no way set apart from the rest of the children in the family. One should encourage the members of the household to take this attitude. Self-pity, which comes from an over-emphasis of a difficulty, has an unfavourable influence upon personality development. Human beings are often thoughtless and unintentionally cruel toward handicapped persons, who desire nothing so much as to be received on an equal footing, and to be made to feel that they are in no way set apart from the rest of the group because of their handicap. Children should not be allowed to mimic, ridicule or to impose upon a deaf child. It is because of society's attitude towards him, primarily, that the deaf person often becomes morose, unsocial, super-sensitive and moody about his limitations, and

[1] Nitchie, E. B., *Lip Reading*, 1912.

then it is possible that he will fail to make the best use of his special abilities, because of the inferiority feelings which have taken a firm hold upon him.

It is not surprising that deaf children should develop " temper-tantrums " in certain situations. It must often appear to them that adults deal with them very stupidly and unsympathetically. Mothers might assist in the early development of the deaf child by establishing an earlier contact with some of the special schools or special teachers for the deaf, before the child is old enough to attend special classes or to go to a special school. The nursery-school movement might well be extended to include the specially handicapped child, while he is still of the plastic school age.

One finds in the literature among teachers of speech correction, speech pathologists, otologists and clinicians, much difference of opinion as to the possibility of improving auditory acuity by training. Ewing has found, with his students, that by raising the intensity of sounds used above the level of their threshold at different intensities, he is able to improve the acuity in both adults and children in many cases.[1] This is also in agreement with the findings of Fröschels.[2] Ewing reports that the majority of his test cases were those in which deafness was congenital or hereditary. He found that deafness in the remaining cases which he selected for study was the result of meningitis, measles, whooping-cough, convulsions, aphasia, concussions and middle-ear infections. His patients tended to confuse both consonant and vowel sounds, in high-frequency deafness, and the *u, e, o* and *a* sounds were therefore often confused and words containing these vowels were misread or misunderstood.[3]

[1] Ewing, A. W. G., *Aphasia in Children*, p. 74.

[2] Fröschels, E., *Kindersprache und Aphasie*, 1918, pp. 40–42.

[3] Ewing, A. W. G., *Aphasia in Children*, pp. 41–51.

NOTE.—Crandall of the Bell Telephone Company found that the average pitch used by women whom he tested was near middle C, or 256 cycles per second. The male voice is lower pitched and is of a different vibration rate, due to structural differences in the larynxes of men and women.

His deviations from norms, in high-frequency deafness, he found to be due primarily to differences in auditory sense organs, and only secondarily to non-auricular factors such as motor, intellectual or emotional components. There was no significant difference between men and women in his tests, and he found that matters of health had a higher correlation with variability in hearing, than had the latter with Chronological Age.

## ALALIA PHYSIOLOGICA

This form of dyslalia is due to no organic disorder, but rather to rate of development. It is " physiologic ", rather than organic, being characterized by temporary mutism in infancy, and by delay in learning to talk. We have touched briefly upon the absence of speech in such cases, in the opening chapter. We shall now consider it as it occurs in children who develop slowly, and in whom normal speech appears somewhat later than in the average child. The backward child is not necessarily mentally deficient, even though he is usually educationally retarded at the outset. We even find a description of delayed development in the histories of a number of eminent men.[1] It appears more frequently in boys than in girls, according to literature.

The retarded child may begin to talk before the age of three, but considerably later than the average child. By the time he begins to go to school his speech may be up to the average. The chief danger in such delay lies in the fact that it tends to make it more difficult for a child to catch up with the better socialized child who has learned to talk earlier. It also affects the personality unfavourably, tending to make a child conscious of his backwardness or inability to cope successfully with other children of his age. Excessive timidity, effeminacy and unsocial conduct may result. It is sometimes impossible

---

[1] Darwin, Edison, Newton, Scott and Sheridan developed very slowly as children, showing few indications of that genius which later brought distinction.

to tell whether a child is *unable* to talk, or only poorly socialized.  His infancy may have been unduly prolonged due to the home environment—some unfortunate habit, such as enuresis, may have caused him to feel inferior. In such cases the teacher and the parent should co-operate in seeking medical advice.

When a child is held back or inhibited by an unsatisfactory environment, his speech may fail to develop at the usual period.  Moreover, if there is no social urge, no social requirement for speech, the child may prolong the infantile period of utter dependence, especially if adults anticipate his needs and desires so as to render articulate speech unnecessary.  The child whose mental processes function at a low level due to lack of stimulation or due to lack of innate intelligence, is often dull and backward, and is found to acquire speech habits more slowly than does the average child.  In such cases a physical examination is usually given to ascertain whether or not there is any organic cause for the delay ; the family history and the child's environment are also carefully scrutinized to find out whether or not they show any reason for the child's slow progress.

### ALALIA PROLONGATA

We have made reference to this difficulty in the first chapter, under speech development of infancy.  We shall discuss it here, because the prolongation of infantile speech habits affects the development of normal speech habits not only in early childhood, but sometimes remains as a hang-over or an infantile fixation into much later years.  The delay or perseverance may have an obscure psychic explanation, with no physiological basis, so far as can be determined.  We will briefly summarize the speech development of a child of this type.

### *Case of Jimmy*

Jimmy was a child of four years, living on a large dairy farm.  He was well cared for physically, but had no playmates.   His father was always occupied with the supervision of the farm, and his mother was busily engaged in the dairy much of the time.   Jimmy's only companion was a maid, who usually had other work to do, while she was "keeping an eye" on Jimmy.   She was a good servant, but knew little about children, and so Jimmy lacked mental stimulation and showed the effect of too little active interest and exercise in the pursuits of childhood.   Everybody neglected him mentally.

When tested by the psychologist Jimmy was found to be of normal intelligence, according to performance tests. He responded to no tests involving language, but made a good score on the Pintner-Patterson tests.   His hearing was found to be fairly acute, when roughly measured, and he was able to make a few speech sounds, since he did this spontaneously, although not responding directly to any of the linguistic tests.   The medical examination was negative.   A study of the family situation revealed that Jimmy's negative reactions to speech stimuli were due to environmental factors which had fostered a natural slowness in learning to talk.   The father had also been delayed in speech development as compared with other children in his family.

It was recommended by the speech specialist and the psychologist that Jimmy should be given playmates— preferably other children near his own age—that he be allowed pet animals, and that the mother herself should give more time to fostering his speech development by direct stimulation through pictures, plays, games, object-lessons, and the like.   In due time he did learn to talk, but at last accounts had not yet made up for the early retardation, either in speech acquisition or in socialization, as compared with the average child.

## Case of Ellen

Ellen was the only child of parents who anticipated her slightest wish.   She received more attention, without attempting to speak, than do most children who talk.

What wonder, then, that she found it most profitable to remain silent ? She was four years of age when first brought to the speech teacher. She was found to be normal in intelligence and her hearing was good. Physician and teacher agreed that her retardation was due to influences within the home environment, and not to any physiological difficulty or disorder. The mother was given instructions and suggestions for the speech re-education of the child, and was told that progress would very likely depend upon home co-operation. After some weeks of instruction, Ellen talked very well.

## Socialization

A child who has been well socialized at home, rarely shows undue timidity or maladjustment in school. If an only child has lacked the opportunity to play with other children, or if there is a great discrepancy between the ages of the youngest child and his next older brother or sister, the child may be more infantile, or less well socialized than one with many playmates near his own age, one from a large family, or from a better socialized home.

Observations made by workers in schools show us that it requires the expenditure of a vast amount of tact, time and energy on the part of the kindergarten teacher to draw an unsocial child into the group activities, so as to become well-socialized. The quality of his speech utterances during this period have considerable diagnostic value for the teacher and the psychologist, because of the light which they shed upon the home situation. The backward child, the timid or awkward child may be at a considerable disadvantage in starting school life, because of poor socialization at home. Stimulating a child to normal social participation in his little group, encouraging him in speech activity, would seem to be a part of the pre-school development desirable for every normal child, and in this his mother may become the chief teacher and director. The responsibility for the child's social attitude when he enters school rests very largely upon the home.

## BARYLALIA or CLUTTERING [1, 2]

Of these two terms, the first more nearly corresponds to the medical description ; a second or more popular term is also given. In such speech there is a noticeable clumsiness or indistinctness in utterance. It is not uncommon in a child who already possesses another handicap in addition to a speech defect. It may consist in the dropping of letters or syllables and is usually characterized as hasty speech.

Such speech is often found in high-strung, over-reacting or over-stimulated children of the pre-school age as well as among older children and adults. Fröschels describes it as one of the preliminary stages in stuttering. The speech may remain merely " cluttered " and without developing a true stutter, or it may pass on to the development of stuttering in which less speed in utterance is apparent.[3] " Clutterers " are often children of excellent mentality. They are rapid thinkers, rapid reacting generally, and the speech is only a symptom of excessively rapid mental processes which outrun the motor speech mechanism by too great a margin. The speech becomes chaotic, jerky, unrhythmic, and often incoherent.

Speech of this type is found among adults, as well as in children, and is usually the result of intense emotional strain, anxiety, fear, neurasthenia or an overwrought nervous state having its origin in unconscious dreads and fears, or in extreme tension under which the individual habitually exists. The speaker may be quite unaware of the existence of the fears, tension, and cluttered speech. During the World War cases of cluttering were found, which were akin to stuttering and to various mental

[1] Wolfe, W. B., *Hygeia*, 5, 273, Je. '27, " The Bridge of Speech."

[2] Erskine, J., *Nation*, 120 : 410–411, Apr. 1925, " Do Americans speak English."

[3] This type of speech is described in the German literature of Gutzmann, Leibmann and Nadoleczny, and has been described by Fröschels in *Kindersprache und Aphasie*, 1918.

disorders which led to hysteria, phobias, obsessions and other disturbed states. The difficulty often cleared up, at least temporarily, when the patient was removed to a new environment or when therapeutic measures were employed. Frequently the mere uncovering of the mental state which was at the basis of the disorder enabled the patient to dispel his anxiety and to clear up his speech difficulty.[1]

We have purposely digressed from the study of speech in childhood to the disturbances of a similar nature found among adults, because we know very little as yet about the psychic causes and neurotic bases for fears of childhood which lead to speech disturbances. Much useful knowledge has been gained within the last few years as a result of the study of a large number of speech disturbances which occurred during the Great War, many of which resemble closely some of the common speech disorders of childhood.[2]

Conditions which are unfavourable to normal emotional stability, the teasing of a child by older brothers or sisters or by a nagging parent, are sufficient to interfere with the development of a normal personality. The child may find the effort to secure some degree of independence of action so great, that he cannot attain it without undue strain and nervousness, because of adult interference and thwarting of his little strivings for independence. In order to get a hearing at all, he may have to speak with great rapidity to prevent interruption, and especially in order to make himself heard before he can be thwarted by adults in the family. Fear of censure or blame may cause him to speak rapidly, or may instead foster a timid, hesitant or uncertain utterance. Eventually this becomes a part of his personality, and his habitual way of reacting.

It is not to be wondered at that speaking often and repeatedly under unfavourable conditions should account for the failure of many children to attain clear speech. The wonder is that they are aggressive enough to attain

---

[1] Culpin, Millais, *Medicine and the Man*, 1927, chs. 1-2.
[2] Southard, *Shellshock and Neuropsychiatry*, 1919.

as much skill as they do in this difficult performance, which demands both dexterity and mental concentration. Parents do not usually feel much concern, until a child passes from the cluttered, chaotic stage into an actual stutter. They are fortunate if the child clears up his difficulty without it being set through becoming conscious. The adult is sometimes responsible for " setting " the habit in the child's mind by constant nagging, scolding or ridicule. This is bound to retard not only the clearing up of the difficulty, but is liable to exercise an unfavourable influence upon the personality of the child as well.

Tredgold [1] speaks of the unstable child of undue irritability, suggestibility and neurotic tendencies, whose mind becomes unbalanced so that extraordinary behaviour results. There is also a marked disturbance in personality present. Cluttered speech is one of the early indications of imbalance which one often finds in such children.

Clutterers are often found in families where one or more adults have rapid, jerky, tense or unrhythmic speech. It is not strange that a child should copy models of speech as of other modes of behaviour. Imitation plays a large part in his growth and development, whether the model imitated be good or bad. The child lacks the discernment of adults in selecting what he shall imitate. He imitates quite spontaneously a lisp, a stutter, or rapid, jerky utterance, if he hears them frequently enough, and if no counter-tendency is set up by better models or by training in better speech.

The principal of a private school was much shocked to find that his small boy of three years was acquiring an astonishing vocabulary of profanity which he took great pride in " trying out " on the family on all sorts of occasions. This child was in the period of rapid speech learning, when he most readily acquired new and unusual sounds by imitation, regardless of meanings. He was fascinated with the new words he heard used on the baseball field, and not only stored up these words, but

[1] Tredgold, *Lectures*, Central Association for Mental Welfare, July, 1931 ; Tredgold, *Mental Deficiency*, 1918. (See Index *re* Speech.)

D

immediately applied them himself, as though to ascertain their meaning by the conduct of the adults who heard them. He apparently enjoyed the effect produced on adults, when he used his new vocabulary. Punishment seemed to be of no avail. Very wisely the parents ceased to appear shocked at the child's utterances. Sometimes they calmly corrected him by saying the sentence over without the undesirable epithet, at other times they simply ignored the matter. After a short time this stage in the child's speech development settled itself, and the undesirable words ceased to appear. This boy was not a " naughty " or perverse child, but on the contrary gave promise of brilliancy and precocity. His accidental speech habits were due to environment in playtime, and to a good memory and an active brain.

Clearing up cluttered, excessively rapid speech in children who learn by example should be comparatively simple, if one could secure the full co-operation of parents. Few adults will take the necessary time and forethought to improve their own utterance in order to help the child. Mothers usually respond better than fathers in this regard, but fathers regard niceties of speech as particularly woman's realm, and often scorn to take an interest in improving their own speech habits. We have already called attention to the fact that it is much more difficult to alter the speech of adults than of children.

When a parent is willing to co-operate, the best aid to good speech is a good example in the home, and one sees no reason why mother and teacher may not work together to aid the child's speech development. It is more economical than to send the child to a teacher each day. Speech clinics are not always available.

The parental model which is desirable for the child should perhaps be explained, as we do not wish to imply that parents should adopt an over-precise, artificially careful manner of speaking. Such speech is not natural and is not a good example. The parents should strive to speak clearly, naturally, calmly, in as effortless a manner as possible, and with reasonably well-modulated tones.

Harsh, strident tones; hoarse, abrupt tones; high-pitched, nervous, whining, or complaining speech which approaches nagging; and too much " mouthing " of words is far from being a good example for the young child.

If a mother can succeed in arousing the interest of the child in games and plays, through the use of toy animals and coloured picture-books, making one's own speech-scrap-book, as the writer does, with young children, it will aid the child in the initiation of desirable speech habits and in the elimination of undesirable ones. A brief weekly check-up with the speech teacher may be all that is required. For this reason it is well that the mother should be present for at least a part of the speech lesson, when the child goes to his teacher, in order to understand what is being done and in order to success-fully follow up the work at home. Mothers are close to the emotional life of the child, and feel so keenly the child's errors and deviations, that they sometimes prevent, when they most desire to *aid* progress. When a mother finds it hard to be reasonably objective in dealing with her own child, she should be urged to take up some work in mental hygiene or in child psychology in order that she may take a less subjective attitude, and be less emotional and personal in dealing with her offspring.

In cities where child guidance clinics are established, there is often a worker in speech pathology, or speech correction. A mother should endeavour to consult some-one with training in speech disorders, or should discuss the matter with a physician or a clinical worker who is familiar with this field, as early as possible in the history of the speech disturbance. The longer one delays, the firmer the grip which the undesirable speech habits may take. The longer the habits are allowed to persist, the more difficult it will be to eradicate them, except in unusual cases.

### IDIOLALIA

This is a form of dyslalia characterized by the sub-stitution of unusual and inaccurate sounds for vowels and consonants, so that the language appears to be un-intelligible ; the same sound or combination of sounds is always used to express the same idea, however. Many refer to it as idioglossia or invented language.[1]

Tredgold mentions idioglossia as a type of speech defect often found in dull or backward children and in the mentally deficient. It is also found in children in whom there is a neuropathic taint, and whose history gives evidence of retardation, physical or mental, in infancy. These children are often highly unstable and erratic. They may develop an " individual language ", intelligible to some other small child in the family perhaps, or to the mother, but unintelligible to anyone else. Such children, if allowed to follow their own inclinations, may delay acquisition of the language of their family for several years. Progress in speech is then much more difficult than when earlier efforts are made to break up infantile or individualistic language development and to replace it with the desired language habits.

The occurrence of such speech in three pairs of twins, with whom the writer has worked, gave evidence of unfavourable mental and physical development in infancy as well as unfortunate physical or mental hereditary influences which seemed to foster a neuropathic tendency in each case, and to engender emotional instability. The speech, however, was not so unintelligible as previous reports of such special " languages " would lead us to believe. A shorthand transcription of their words and sentences showed that all three sets of twins possessed one characteristic in common. They were found to be dropping or mutilating initial, middle and final consonants, and sometimes to be modifying the root vowel. In some instances they gave the vowels in the correct sequence and quite clearly, but simply substituted a lip movement such as *p*, *b* or *m* for more difficult or less frequent consonants. They gave *p*, *b* and *m* sounds in some positions in many words, but rarely attempted *t*, *d*, *n*, *ng*, *s*, *r*, *l*, *k* and *g*. If attempted at all, these sounds usually gave

---

[1] Tredgold, *Mental Deficiency*, pp. 128, 416.

way to substitutions, while such sounds as *zh*, *ch*, *j* and *th* were not even attempted.  MacCarthy [1] also reports some speech difficulties which seems to agree with our findings, in pairs of twins whom she studied in connection with her work at the University of Minnesota.

It is possible that many of the idiolalias are more closely patterned after actual speech sounds than we have hitherto imagined.  The speech of babyhood is frequently unintelligible to adults, and without careful phonetic analysis it is impossible, usually, to tell immediately whether the child's speech bears any resemblance to the speech of his environment or not.  When such sounds are unintelligible and yet seem to be used very definitely by the child as word symbols, having a constant meaning, they should be transcribed as accurately as possible, with a view to analysis and psychological study, as this will not only aid in understanding the nature of the difficulty, but will also serve to direct the teacher who is to undertake the matter of speech correction.

## PARALALIA—LISPING

This form of dyslalia means the production of a distinctly different sound from that desired, or the constant substitution of one sound for another.[2]  The common term used in the literature to describe such speech is *lisping*.  Scripture [3] uses the term stammering to cover the entire field of letter-substitutions and lisps, and many writers make a further distinction between them by referring to the sound-substitution made for the letter itself, as, *rhotacism* for difficulty on the *r* sounds ; *lambdacism* for difficulty with *l* sounds ; *sigmatism* for difficulty with *s* sounds ; but we believe that this is too complicated for ordinary use, and therefore recommend the term *paralalia* as the best descriptive term, and *lisping* as the term for more common use.

[1] MacCarthy, Dorothy, *Language and Speech Development*, 1930.
[2] Robbins-Stinchfield, *Dictionary of Terms Dealing with Disorders of Speech*, p. 18.
[3] Scripture, E., *Stuttering and Lisping*, 1920.

When the child says, "Iss 'oo doin' det me a 'itoo fis'?" instead of, "Are you going to get me a little fish?" the adult is at first merely amused and often enjoys talking to the child in its own vernacular. The perseverance of such speech for months or years, however, becomes rather less amusing. To the writer it is rather appalling that such numbers of adults are encountered every day in any city or town, who have failed to eliminate some of the infantile speech habits which should have been overcome in the pre-school period, and which have persisted until it has permanently marred the enunciation, as adult speech habits do not readily change. It is natural and normal for all children to give some letter-substitutions in learning to talk, but there should be rapid improvement even during the pre-school years, and any normal child should be able to talk plainly by the time he is ready for school, and should by this time have eliminated most of the letter-substitutions and speech inaccuracies of infancy.

Persistence in the mutilation or substitution of one sound for another makes it harder for the child to unlearn the wrong habits. It is not always entirely corrected in adulthood, and even in college one finds occasionally some girl who has no *r* or *l* in her vocabulary, but who substitutes instead the lip sound of *w*. A little guidance in childhood might very easily have overcome this speech inaccuracy. Such corrections are much more easily accomplished with small children within the home environment, if done without calling undue attention to the child's speech deficiencies. Tongue-tie rarely occurs, and is not usually the reason for letter-substitutions, despite some statements often made to the contrary.

One of the most helpful ways of gaining a child's co-operation in improving speech habits, is to take an ordinary blank-book in a fairly strong binding, and to cut out pictures of objects representing all of the speech sounds in our language. These pictures may be pasted in the notebook, and the names may be printed in the margin, together with word-lists illustrative of the desired sounds. The child becomes interested in making his own speech-book, and this aids him in the development of language habits. As he eliminates faults and gives a correct sound to replace the old substitution, we sometimes place a kindergarten star on the page of his book, to remind him to continue to make the correction and to denote our approval of his efforts and to stimulate him to further endeavour. Incidentally, this method, borrowed from the habit-clinics of Massachusetts, is a very useful one to employ in work with deaf or crippled children, as the play-spirit involved and approval given, interests and entertains the child more than does unrewarded effort or unmotivated behaviour and ordinary speech drill.

## SPECIAL METHODS

The five speech-learning habits mentioned by Palmer [1] are very useful in training children to overcome letter-substitutions, lisping and minor speech difficulties. They are :—

### 1. *Auditory Imitation*

This is learning based on auditory observation. Children who are poor in auditory learning may often be taught by the visual look-and-say method.

### 2. *Oral Imitation*

Following the auditory observation, the child must learn to say orally the sounds which he has heard. He also observes circumstances under which the words are used and learns when to apply them. Neglect of observation and imitation are mentioned as one of the primary causes of language difficulty in children and in adults.

### 3. *Catenizing*

This involves making the necessary co-ordination of successive movements. The motions must be made habitual by practice. Sounds difficult for adults are not difficult for children, before the ages of fourteen or fifteen

[1] Palmer, H. E., *The Five Speech-Learning Habits*, 1923.

years.  Young children must learn by rote certain sounds and words.  This may be done through poetry, rhymes, proverbs, short prose selections and stories.

#### 4. *Semanticizing*

This means to fuse the word to its meaning.  Children are also keener at this process than are adults.  It must be done for words, phrases, and for entire sentences.

#### 5. *Composition by Analogy*

Grammar is not the best way to teach a language, according to Palmer, but through the direct method of usage comes correctness of form, knowledge of structure, inflection and decision.  Conversations, changing from active to passive, and correction of the child's mistakes as they occur will enable him soon to use the language successfully for himself.

### REFERENCES

*Archives of Otology.*
Best, H., *The Deaf*, N.Y., 1914, p. 324.
Bruhn, Martha, *Muller Waller Method of Lip-Reading*, Boston.
Bunch, C. C., *Measurement of Acuity of Hearing*, Psycho. Monog., 1922, p. 69.
Census Reports : *Report on the Insane, Feeble-minded, Deaf and Blind.*
Clarke School for the Deaf, Northampton, Mass., *Reports and Bulletins.*
Central Inst. for the Deaf, St. Louis, *Reports.*
Davenport, C. B., *Heredity in Relation to Eugenics*, 1911.
Ewing, A. W. G., *Aphasia in Children*, London, 1928.
Ewing, Irene E., *Lip-Reading.*
Fröschels, E., *Kindersprache und Aphasie*, 1918.
Galton, Francis, *Natural Inheritance*, 1889.
*International Record of Charities and Corrections*, 1886–1931.
*Jour. of Amer. Medical Association*, 1909–1931.
*Jour. of British Medical Association*, 1900–1931.
Keller, Helen, *The World I Live In.  The Story of My Life.*
Marsden, O. C., *Training for Efficiency*, N.Y.
Nitchie, E. B., *Lip-Reading*, N.Y., 1912.
*N.Y. Med. Jour.*, I, 1889–1931.
*Proceedings of the N.E.A.*, 1901–1931.
*Proceed. of the Internat. Otolog. Congress*, IX, 1913.
*Proceed. of the National Association of the Deaf*, 1912–1931.

# COMMON SPEECH DIFFICULTIES 57

*Proceed. of the Amer. Association to Promote Teaching of Speech to the Deaf*, IV, 1894.
*Volta Review*, Washington, D.C.
Wright, John D., Oral School for the Deaf, N.Y., *Reports and Bulletins*, 1900–1931.

### In Literature

Wallace, Lew, *Prince of India*.
Turgenev, *The Mute*.

# CHAPTER IV

## COMMON SPEECH DIFFICULTIES OF CHILDHOOD
### (*continued*): DYSLALIA AND DYSPHEMIA

(*a*) URANOSCHISMATICA OR CLEFT-PALATE SPEECH
(*b*) DYSLALIA AND DYSPHEMIA IN BLIND CHILDREN

1. *American Schools for the Blind*
2. *Austrian Schools for the Blind* (*Vienna*)

DYSLALIA has been defined as a speech defect of organic
or of functional origin, dependent upon malformation or
imperfect innervation of the tongue, soft palate or other
organs of articulation. The speech is impaired due to
the condition of the external speech organs. It may
range from a mild lisp to rapid, cluttered speech ; it may
be associated with deafness, or with physiologic or organic
conditions which are unfavourable to normal speech
development ; the beginning of learning to talk may have
been so delayed that speech retardation and persistence of
infantile speech habits continue far beyond the early
infancy period ; children may invent a language of their
own, manifesting what is called " idioglossia ". There is
another form of dyslalia which is called rhinolalia-aperta
or uranoschismatica, as in cleft-palate speech.[1] Uranoschismatica, or cleft-palate speech, is characterized by
thick, breathy or nasal utterance in which all speech
sounds except the nasals have become modified, and in
which plosives and vowels become nasal sounds. The
longer term is the more accurate as a description, but the
popular term is cleft-palate speech. Short-palate speech

[1] Robbins-Stinchfield, *Dictionary of Terms Dealing with Disorders of
Speech.*

PLATE I

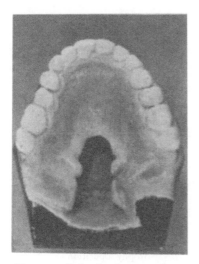

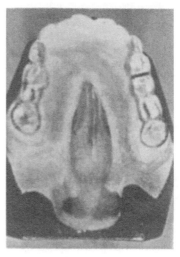

Type 1. Cleft of soft palate above      Type 2. Cleft of hard and soft palate

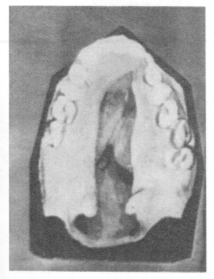

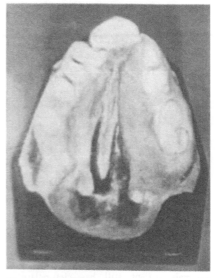

Type 3. Simple harelip and complete cleft      Type 4. Double harelip and complete cleft

VARIOUS TYPES OF CLEFT PALATE AND HARELIP

*(The photographs from which these studies were made were kindly given by Dr. John J. Fitzgibbon, Holyoke, Mass.)*

[face p. 58

PLATE II

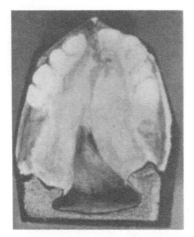

Type 5. Incomplete closure, following complete cleft-palatal operation

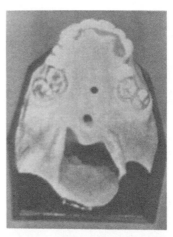

Type 6. Perforation following Brophy operation

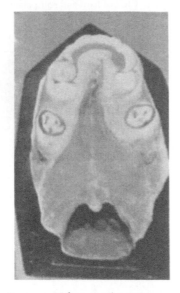

Type 7. Velum so short that upon repair patient still has cleft-palate speech in spite of closure of cleft

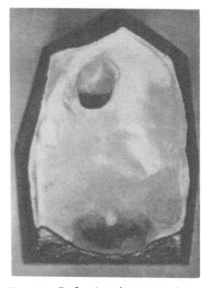

Type 8. Perforation due to carcinoma. Similar condition is often found in syphilitic lesion

*(Courtesy of Dr. J. Fitzgibbon)*

shows similar characteristics, the speech sometimes being affected by the velar insufficiency.[1]

The resonance, quality and articulation found in normal speech are modified in the cleft-palate patient. Most surgeons feel that the cleft should be closed at about the age of two years, or before speech habits have been acquired or set to any great extent. Some writers assert that it is nearly impossible to secure normal speech in the case of adults, following a closure of the cleft, as the muscular development of the throat and palatal region differs from that of the normal throat, and the nerve supply may be altered, following operative surgery ; these writers believe that it is more difficult to unlearn habits of speech in adulthood, than at an earlier age. For this reason, as well as for other reasons, mainly physiological, early operative procedure is recommended, wherever the cleft is narrow enough to permit of improvement through surgery. When the cleft is too wide for satisfactory surgical results, the wearing of an obturator or palatal appliance is usually recommended.

The causes of cleft-palate condition are not definitely known. Theories vary widely from the superstition that a child born with a cleft palate is " marked " by some prenatal maternal impression or injury, to a more recent theory that toxic substances in the maternal blood-stream may interfere with the embryonic development. Unsuccessful attempts at abortion have also been given by some writers as a possible cause.[2] Studies of thirty-two jaguars born with cleft palates, in one of the zoos, revealed that in this case the probable cause was malnutrition. The mother bore a litter of twenty-five normal cubs when she was fed a balanced food ration.[3]

Fitzgibbon[4] holds that unsuccessful contraceptive measures may interfere with the normal development

[1] Federspiel, M., *Harelip and Cleft Palate*, 1927.
Additional references : Blair and Ivy, *Essentials of Oral Surgery* ; Case, Calvin, *Dental Orthopedia and Correction of Cleft Palate*.
[2] Fitzgibbon, J. J., *Congenital Cleft Palate*.
[3] Federspiel, M., *ibid*.
[4] Fitzgibbon, J. J., *loc. cit*.

of the fœtus, the palatal processes failing to fuse, as a result. Heredity certainly seems to play an important part in the incidence of palatal cleft, as it has been found to occur for several generations in some family stocks.[1]

We are less concerned with the physiology of cleft palate and theories of causative factors, than with the actual speech conditions which accompany it. The cleft may be unilateral or double. It may be accompanied by harelip, and the cleft may be complete, through both of these structures, or may be partial, extending only for a short distance. When harelip is present the mouth and lips are deformed, nursing is difficult, and malnutrition becomes one of the chief reasons for early operative procedure. There may be only a tiny opening into the nasal passage, or the fissure may be so wide and deep that the turbinates are plainly visible from the oral cavity.

The physiological dangers of cleft-palatal condition through malnutrition have been mentioned. There is also the danger of infection within the nasal cavities, due to regurgitation of food and to the exposure of the nasal passage to substances entering the mouth. In addition to this, the speech is affected to a greater or less extent, according to the nature of the cleft, the results of operative surgery which has been employed, the flexibility of the muscles in the glosso-pharyngeal region, and their ability to constrict or to compensate for the loss of the soft palate, by constricting or closing off the nasal from the oral cavity, during the production of speech sounds. Only three English sounds should be nasalized, viz., *n, m,* and *ng*.

Operative surgery is employed when a closure may be effected which will give sufficient flexibility to the structures involved in articulation, to aid in the production of oral resonance, and to prevent undue nasal resonance. A good operative *closure*, however, does not insure good

[1] Rosanoff, A., *Unpublished Lectures.* Research studies of twins in United States and Canada, by Rosanoff, yet all indicate that heredity is the primary factor, as they find many cases of cleft palate in monozygotic twins, showing that the anomaly must have been present in the germ plasm in these cases.

PLATE III

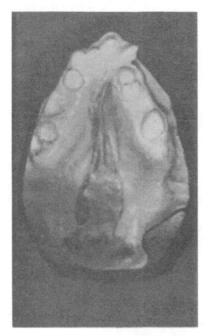

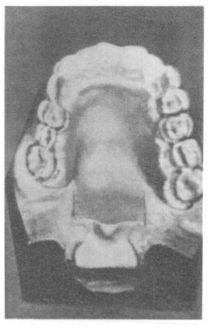

Type 9. Typical malocclusion of cleft palate case. Type of malocclusion often found in torsi-version to median line

Type 10. Position of bulb of Fitzgibbon palatal appliance, irrespective of type of case

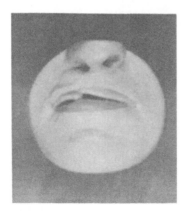

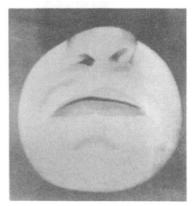

Type 11. Harelip. Appearance of patient when first seen

Type 12. Same patient, following operation

*(Courtesy of Dr. John Fitzgibbon)*

PLATE IV

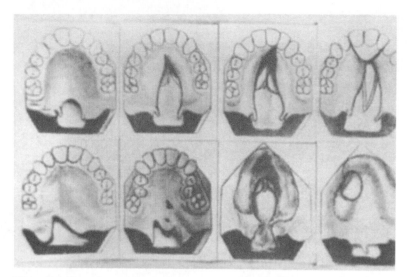

Type 13. Grouping together of the various types of palatal cleft shown above

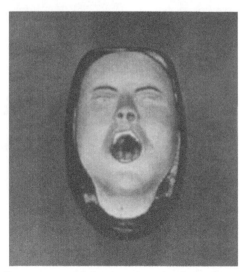

Type 14. From wax model showing view of typical complete cleft palate

*(Courtesy of Dr. J. J. Fitzgibbon)*

[ face p. 61

*speech*, if the control of the velum and of the pharyngeal muscles is so inadequate as to make it impossible to secure the necessary action of the glosso-pharyngeal muscles and the constrictors of the pharynx. The patient must be taught the control of these muscles, through much practice, and the surgical procedure in itself is not sufficient to restore normal speech. " Gargling " or exercise of the palatal muscles, and gentle massage are often used.[1]

When the cleft is too wide or too deep to be successfully closed by means of the bone-flap, by wire ligatures and the transfer of soft tissue, the use of an obturator is recommended, but the size, shape and general features of these vary greatly. The ideal one is that which gives the patient immediate improvement in the production of speech sounds, and which enables him, after a few lessons, to speak with little or no excess nasality. It is often necessary to modify whatever obturator is used, both at the outset and at frequent intervals during its use. This is determined by the physician, when the patient appears for examination from time to time. The phonographic record of his speech, or even an ordinary dictaphone may help both patient and doctor in eliminating undesirable speech noises, and in developing the correct speech sounds. The author has heard immediate improvement in the speech of patients following the insertion of two different types of obturators. One is that made by an American dentist,[2] and the second is a European appliance.[3] Both have been demonstrated abroad with success.

### Effect of this Handicap upon the Personality of the Growing Child

It is especially important to attend to the closure of the palate in early childhood if possible, while speech habits are plastic and not too difficult to modify. If the

---

[1] Children's Hospital, Chicago, massage method.

[2] Fitzgibbon, J. J., Holyoke, Mass., Fitzgibbon appliance.

[3] Speech Clinic, University of Vienna, Fröschels-Schalitt appliance.

cleft is neglected until the child is of school age, his companions soon notice the peculiarity in his utterance and are liable to make him very self-conscious. The child then suffers the pangs of inferiority and hypersensitivity, and becomes unhappy and unsocial, unless he happens to be unusually aggressive, or above average in intelligence and in socialization. The more intelligent the child, the more sensitive he may be. However, the factor of intelligence is important in speech training, as such children, with good auditory discrimination and power of concentration easily master the difficulty, following a successful operation or with the aid of an appliance.

Speech workers find that the most rapid progress is made in overcoming rhinolalia by brighter children and by adults. Dull or retarded children and those with poor auditory imagery require a longer training period for the elimination of the excessive nasality. The teacher should endeavour in every way to make the child attempt to accept the fact of his handicap in a natural, objective way, rather than to allow him to make a " crutch " of his handicap, to the detriment of his personality. Hypersensitivity and self-pity or inferiority feelings tend to make either a weakling or a tyrant of any individual, and to foster the hang-over into adult years of infantile mechanisms and behaviour.

The introspections of adult cleft-palatal patients on this point are pertinent, as they tend to show quite clearly that it is hypersensitivity and asocial conduct which have been the greatest detriments to them in adult social adjustments and often in their chosen careers, particularly when it involved speech-making, or the forming of social contacts.

### Speech Disorders among Blind Children

We discussed the speech of the deaf child in an earlier chapter. We wish to spend some little time in the discussion of the speech of another type of specially handicapped child, the blind. Our own speech surveys in schools for the blind revealed not only some of the dysphemias but also a small number of additional speech disorders, following our classification. We find all of these defects also in public school children, but it is our belief that children who suffer from a defect or from deprivation in one of the special senses, are more prone to acquire a speech defect than are children without such a special handicap.

The question of the relation of the blind child to certain disorders of speech is important, because usually such speech defects are remedial, and the prognosis is much better than in the case of the deaf child. Frequently it is also better than in the case of the crippled child, in whom certain muscles associated with speech may be involved in paralysis or injury, and limit the possibility of attaining normal speech. This is often the case with children who have had spastic paralysis, and who never attain normal speech.

The fact of blindness itself is a sufficient handicap, without further limitations, and it is therefore advisable to remove speech defects, whenever they occur in a blind child, as in this way a personality handicap may be removed or prevented, the child's social adjustment may be improved, and his chances for a good economic and social adjustment increased. Even though the blind adult may not be wholly self-supporting, it is desirable that he should be so educated that his personality and capacities may be developed as far as possible.

We often find defects of speech, not only in those suffering from total blindness, but also in those with partial vision. Only about one-tenth of all blind individuals are under twenty years of age; and it is this group, still of school age, with whom we are primarily concerned.

## Legal Aspects of Blindness

Legally, the blind are held to be as strictly accountable for their acts as seeing persons, and they therefore frequently fail to recover damages in case of accident. The lack of vision often causes them to become unusually acute on the auditory side, and on this and on cutaneous impressions they depend to a very great extent for the major part of their education. It is important that speech sounds should be perceived and evaluated by them as intended by the speaker, and that they themselves should reduce any unnecessary strain or effort on their part, by being trained to speak clearly and intelligibly.

Recognizing that speech education is an important phase of the education of the blind, a number of the larger schools for the blind in the United States have not only developed speech-training classes on the artistic side, in which children with histrionic ability may participate in dramatic productions, but in several schools there have been established in connection with the psychological work, speech clinic and speech corrective work, following speech surveys made by the author and her assistants.

## Vocational Aspects

Although vision is an absolute necessity in many professions, so that the actual earnings of the blind are economically more limited than are those of the deaf (as fewer occupations are open to the blind), many of them are excellent musicians, good piano-tuners, and teachers of the blind. Some are engaged as home-makers, domestic helpers, private teachers of other blind individuals, or are in occupations which can be carried on in their own homes. Recent investigations indicate that families of the blind are often in poor economic circumstances and this naturally limits the horizon of the children in such families, unless they are given special educational advantages.

## Personality of the Blind Child

It is not lack of vision which the blind person most dislikes, but the lack of independence. He usually resents manifestations of pity, and wishes to be received on a par with seeing persons. This laudable spirit of independence and desire for self-realization should be encouraged by all persons concerned in educating blind

PLATE V

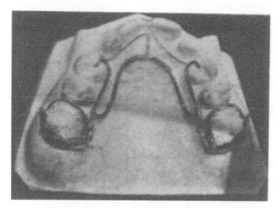

Type 15.   Showing dental appliance which gives
anchorage on the molars

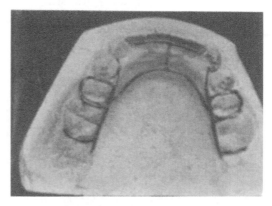

Type 16.   Finger-spring extension for the correction
of malocclusion of another type

TYPICAL DENTAL APPLIANCES USED FOR THE CORRECTION OF MALOCCLUSION

*(Courtesy of " Dental Items of Interest," Brooklyn, N.Y., April 1922)*

[ face p. 64

PLATE VI

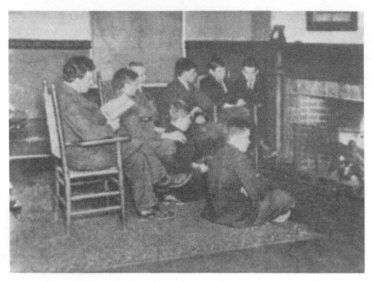

Learning through auditory sensory avenues. Perkins Institution for the Blind, Watertown, Mass.

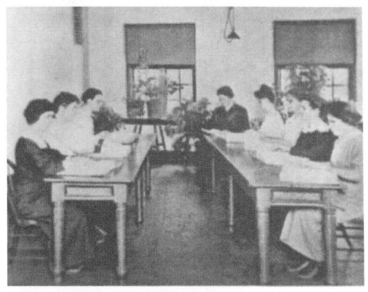

Reading by sense of touch ; training the kinaesthetic and cutaneous sensory avenues. Class in Braille, Perkins Institution children.   The average person becomes too sentimental and creates too great a gulf between himself and the handicapped person.   Popular belief has created a number of superstitions about the blind, such as that they are more spiritual, more docile and childlike than are seeing persons.   We believe this to be an unwarranted assumption. Blind children may be dependent, but not docile ; too trusting in some respects, and unduly suspicious in others ; moody and sensitive ;  but we find these tendencies in seeing children also.   We believe that the social development of the blind child depends quite as much upon the home situation and early environment, physical and social heredity, as is the case with sighted children.   They are neither more precocious and brilliant, nor more stupid and retarded than other children, when given educational advantages or opportunity for normal development.

### Education of the Blind Child

Some States provide special schools for the infant blind.   In others there is usually a kindergarten.   Here we find the best opportunity for the elimination of speech defects, while the child is still plastic and speech habits are not yet set into adult moulds.   Children may usually enter schools for the blind by the age of five years, and there is sometimes a special educational fund, which may be applied to remedial speech training, as is done in the Kindergarten of the Perkins Institution for the Blind, at Watertown, Massachusetts.

The desirability of extending speech training into the upper grades soon becomes apparent.   While speech faults may be eliminated more easily in early childhood, we find in every school a good many children in the upper grades who have not eliminated them, except in schools where the work of speech correction has been under way for a period of years.

### The Speech of the Deaf-blind

The deaf-blind children have received a great deal of time and attention in some cases, especially when they

E

seem fairly precocious, in spite of their double handicap. The voice of the deaf-blind child is generally unpleasant, monotonous and toneless, as is the voice of the deaf-mute who develops speech. Training in speech also enables these doubly handicapped children to overcome depression, timidity, moodiness and discouragement. They may acquire desirable habits of work or study in some field of special interest, through the acquisition of Braille-reading. The correction of remedial handicaps is an important aid to development of personality, for self-expression, for satisfaction in one's social group, and for life adjustment in general. Artistic speech-training for the child who is already well balanced and free from speech handicaps, and speech correction for the child who suffers from personality defect because of the speech difficulty, should both be included in the educational programme in every school for the blind.

### Speech Defects

Any serious physical handicap tends to increase nervous strain, anxiety and the tension under which an individual lives. The specially handicapped child is apt to be most favourably cared for, therefore, in special classes or institutions. Sometimes such handicapped children prove to be exceptionally bright or well socialized and show very little retardation as compared with normal children. Severe competition, awareness of inadequacy to meet various situations, great anxiety and prolonged unsuccessful effort tend to create an unfortunate mental state in handicapped children of any type, and may lead to the onset of a psychoneurosis. Hysteria, neurasthenia, psychasthenia, and serious maladjustment of other types bordering on psychotic states sometimes occur in schools for the blind. When such a condition develops in the already handicapped individual, it intensifies his difficulties considerably, and the prognosis may be less favourable than for a person not suffering with a handicap.[1]

[1] Fladeland, S. V., "Some Psychological Effects of Blindness ", *Journal of Expression*, Boston, 1930.

A study of children by a psychiatrist is often desirable in the schools for the blind, as it is important to discover the cause of the maladjustment as early as possible. Personality defects, associated with speech disorders, have appeared in a number of cases in the schools under our observation.

It is important in special schools to have the co-operation of the medical and dental staff of the institution, as handicapped children have often been physically neglected at home ; and it takes some little time, after their entrance into an institution. The correction of malocclusion, removal of diseased tonsils or adenoids is often an important preliminary to remedial speech work in special schools, just as it is in public school speech clinics.

In the schools for the blind where speech surveys have been made by the author (including all of the children in the Perkins Institution, and in the Pennsylvania Institution for the Blind, and including about half of those in the New York School for the Blind) there were more children found with dyslalia than with any other single type of speech defect. The speech ranged from mild oral inaccuracies and letter substitution, to lateral lisping, sigmatism, and severe oral inaccuracies.

In the two schools for the blind in Vienna in which speech tests were given in German by the writer, dyslalia was found to exceed all other types of speech defects. Spasmophemia or stuttering took second place in the Vienna schools, along with nasality or rhinolalia. Spasmophemia or stuttering took second place in the three American schools. These cases in themselves might fully occupy the time of a teacher of speech correction, even were no other types of speech defect found.

In spasmophemia we have a speech disorder to which children may easily become subject, if for any reason they labour under great nervous strain, tension, fear, depression, or feelings of inferiority. In the schools for the blind we have found not only spasmophemia, but other forms of dysphemia such as hysterical stuttering, voluntary muteness, neurotic lisping, and rapid, cluttered speech,—the speech disturbance being sometimes chronic, but often intermittent or variable.

The results of a speech survey at Perkins Institution are recorded and classified in the following table.

CLASSIFICATION OF SPEECH DEFECTS FOLLOWING SPEECH SURVEY IN PERKINS INSTITUTION FOR THE BLIND, WATERTOWN, MASSACHUSETTS, 220 SUBJECTS [1]

| Type of Speech Difficulty | School where Found | | | | | | | |
|---|---|---|---|---|---|---|---|---|
| | Upper | | Lower | | Kindergarten | | Total | |
| | Girls | Boys | Girls | Boys | Girls | Boys | No. | Per cent. of Group |
| DYSLALIA | | | | | | | | |
| a. Extreme oral inaccuracy | — | 1 | — | — | — | — | 1 | 0·8 |
| b. Letter substitution | 2 | — | 3 | 2 | 4 | 8 | 19 | 15·0 |
| c. Rhinolalia | 3 | — | — | — | — | — | 3 | 2·2 |
| d. Oral inaccuracy and letter substitution | 1 | 1 | 3 | — | — | — | 5 | 4·0 |
| e. Mild oral inaccuracy | 14 | 11 | 10 | 7 | 5 | 6 | 53 | 42·0 |
| f. Barbaralalia (foreign accent) | — | 1 | — | — | 1 | — | 2 | 2·0 |
| g. Oral inaccuracy and lisp | 9 | 3 | 1 | — | 2 | — | 15 | 12·0 |
| h. Deafness and oral inaccuracy | 1 | 1 | — | — | — | — | 2 | 2·0 |
| i. Lateral lisp | — | — | 1 | — | — | — | 1 | 0·8 |
| DYSLOGIA | | | | | | | | |
| a. Speech expressive of emotional uncontrol and marked maladjustment | — | — | 1 | 1 | — | — | 2 | 2·0 |
| b. Eerie, bat-like quality of voice | — | — | — | — | 2 | — | 2 | 2·0 |
| c. Negatively suggestible w. voluntary muteness | 1 | — | — | — | — | — | 1 | 0·8 |
| d. Introverted, over-self-conscious type | 1 | — | — | — | — | — | 1 | 0·8 |

[1] Survey arranged through co-operation of Prof. S. P. Hayes, consulting psychologist.

CLASSIFICATION OF SPEECH DEFECTS—*continued.*

| TYPE OF SPEECH DIFFICULTY | SCHOOL WHERE FOUND | | | | | | | |
|---|---|---|---|---|---|---|---|---|
| | Upper | | Lower | | Kindergarten | | Total | |
| | Girls | Boys | Girls | Boys | Girls | Boys | No. | Per cent. of Group |
| DYSPHASIA *a.* Paraphasia . . | — | — | — | I | — | — | I | 0·8 |
| DYSPHEMIA *a.* Stuttering . . | I | 2 | — | — | 2 | 3 | 8 | 6·0 |
| DYSPHONIA *a.* Vocal defect, hoarse, harsh, etc. (quality) . . | 3 | 2 | — | — | — | — | 5 | 4·0 |
| *b.* Monotonous, subdued, repressed tones . . . | — | I | — | — | — | — | I | 0·8 |
| DYSRHYTHMIA *a.* Pneumaphrasia (breath-grouping) | — | — | 2 | — | — | — | 2 | 2·0 |
| Total . . | 36 | 23 | 21 | II | 16 | 17 | 124 | 100 |

## *Significant Tendencies*

I. Of the total number (220) to whom the speech tests were given at Perkins Institution, 124 showed speech defects ranging from mild to severe. This constituted 56 per cent. of the entire enrolment, a surprisingly high percentage. Of these, 51 cases or 23 per cent. were boys ; 73 cases or 33 per cent. were girls. This is a different ratio from that usually reported in speech surveys, as the ratio of boys to girls is usually 3 to 1. Here we found the ratio to be 3 girls to 2 boys with speech defects. In spasmophemia, or stuttering, however, our ratio was 2 boys to 1 girl. This corresponds more closely to the ratio usually found, especially for stutterers.

II. There were no cases coming under the head of Dysarthria. The chief reason for this is probably the age factor, and the fact that the dysarthrias are usually found with other physical handicaps. Also, it may be that where there is a triple handicap, such as blindness, with other severe physical handicaps, the child has not reached the institution, or has not survived to reach the age for formal education. Moreover, the dysarthrias increase in adulthood, whereas many other types of speech defect decrease or are eliminated by the time one reaches adulthood.

III. There were more dyslalias than any other type of speech defect, among both boys and girls in all the schools for the blind. There were 101 cases of dyslalia at Perkins, or 46 per cent. of the total number examined there. The commonest type of defect was mild oral inaccuracy, which was more frequent among girls than among boys in both the upper and the lower schools. In the kindergarten it was about the same for both sexes. There were 53 cases of mild oral inaccuracy, or 24 per cent. of the total number examined.

IV. Stuttering was found more frequently in the upper school and in the kindergarten, *i.e.* soon after entrance into the school, and again at adolescence, rather than in the intermediate years. It occurred in a ratio of 2 boys to 1 girl. There were 8 cases in all, or 3½ per cent. of the total number examined.

When the findings for Perkins Institution and for the Pennsylvania School for the Blind are combined, the percentage of speech defects found is 49 per cent. or slightly less than that found in the Perkins Institution alone, and slightly more than that found in the Pennsylvania School alone.[1] The slight difference is almost negligible as between the two schools, but the large numbers indicate that speech defects are more common among such specially handicapped children as are found in schools for the blind than in schools for the seeing. We might expect to find this condition in schools for the deaf, but to a less extent in schools for other handi-

---

[1] Stinchfield, S. M., *Speech Pathology*, p. 81.

MEDIAN SCORES OBTAINED BY 156 SUBJECTS IN THE PENNSYLVANIA INSTITUTION FOR THE BLIND, IN THE B–S SPEECH TESTS[1]

| Grade | Artic. Test A | Oral R. Rate | Silent R. Rate | Spontaneous Sp. Rate | Per cent. of Relevant Words | Subjective Rating | Median C.A. | I.Q. |
|---|---|---|---|---|---|---|---|---|
| Kindergarten . . | 93 | omitted | omitted | 120 | 93·5 | — | — | — |
| II . . | 95 | 38 | 22 | 107·5 | 90 | 15 (out of possible 21 pts.) | 10 | 91 |
| III . . | 95 | 72 | 64 | 112 | 90·5 | 15 | 11–5 | 92 |
| IV . . | 95 | 82 | 92 | 118 | 92 | 15 | 15–4 | 100 |
| V . | ← | ← | ← | ← | ← | ← | ← | ← |
| VI . . | → | → | → | → | → | → | → | → |
| VII . | 95 | 82 | 92 | 118 | 92 | 15 | 15–4 | 100 |

Scores represent both boys and girls combined.

[1] The numbers were so small that for Grades IV to VII the median for all four grades was secured, since the median scores for the norms of public school children remain practically constant for these four grades. There was no eighth grade in the school, the next highest class being the first year high school group. This table should be compared with the norms given in Table III, Chapter XII., p. 284, on "Results of Speech Testing, 1922–1931." The Blanton-Stinchfield Speech Tests, prepared in Braille raised print were used. These are obtainable through C. H. Stoelting & Co., Chicago.

capped children.   Its existence indicates the need for
remedial speech training, as we have here a definite,
tangible defect in addition to blindness, and one which is
remedial.

As a result of the speech surveys at the Perkins
Institution, Pennsylvania Institution at Overbrook, Pennsylvania, and a brief survey at the New York School
for the Blind, covering about 50 per cent. of the children,
remedial speech work has been established in these three
of the largest schools for the blind, as a part of the general
rehabilitation programme.   This is not a part of the
expression and auditorium work, but is under the direction
of special teachers trained in speech pathology and
psychology, as well as in the artistic side of speech work.

Perkins has trained many blind-deaf children since
Dr. Samuel Howe showed the way with Laura Bridgman
as pupil.   During the past year a specially trained teacher
has given her entire time to the education of a blind-deaf
pupil, who has become remarkably facile at muscle
reading, and is developing intelligent speech.   It is our
conviction that every residential school for the blind
should provide special teachers for the education of these
doubly-handicapped children, as they require training
and educational facilities which cannot be given by the
regular class-room teachers.   (See Table, p. 71.)

Comparing these results for blind subjects with those
obtained from a larger group of public school subjects
(717), we find that in the articulation test these subjects
are within the range of the median for the larger group,
which is 92 to 96, Grades I to VII.   In Oral Reading they
fall considerably below the norm set for the larger group,
the range in the public school group, Grades II to VII
being from 96 (Grade II) to 174 (in the higher grades).
The range for the Grades II to VII in the blind school
is 38 (Grade II) to 82 (Grade VII).   In the public school
group the range in silent reading extends from 22–96 (in
Grade I) to 138–225 (Grade VII).   In the above group
the silent reading range extends from 22 (Grade II)

and 64 (Grade III) to 92 (Grades IV to VII). The maximum score in the school for the blind is less than half that obtained for the public school group, whose maximum score was 225.

In the public school group the average rate for spontaneous speech in Grade I was 74–120 words a minute. The average for kindergarten children in the school for the blind was 120 words per minute. The scores in spontaneous speech rate for the public school group in Grades II to V was 108–120 words per minute. The subjects in the school for the blind were within this norm, the median for Grade II being 107·5, for Grade III it was 112, and for Grades IV to VII the median was 118 words per minute.

In percentage of relevant words the range for the public school Grades I to VII was 90–96. The median for the blind children was within this range, being 93·5 for the kindergarten, 90 for the Grade II, 90·5 for Grade III and averaging 92 for Grades IV to VII.

In intelligence and in chronological age there were some interesting comparisons. The blind children tested were on an average three years older than children of the same grade in public schools. Comparing the intelligence quotients of the blind children tested, with the figures given for the White House Conference Report,[1] we find that the median I.Q. for stutterers, those with structural articulatory defects, oral inactivities and sound substitutions was 90–100. The intelligence quotient for the children tested in the school for the blind was 91 for Grade I, 92 for Grade III, and it averaged 100 for Grades IV to VII.

With the co-operation of Dr. Emil Fröschels, Director of the Speech Clinic, General Hospital, University of Vienna, a speech survey of all children of school age in two schools for the blind in Vienna, was made by the

[1] White House Conference Reports, *The Handicapped Child*, 1931. Statistical reports unpublished, prepared by West, Travis and Camp, University of Wisconsin and University of Iowa, for the White House Conference Survey.

author with the assistance of Dr. Badzinsky of the Fröschels clinic, in the spring of 1931. The first was a small school of about 60 children and adults, all of whom were from Jewish families. About 30 children took the speech tests adapted for use in German, including all of the German sounds as listed by the International Phonetic Association Alphabet.

Of the 30 children in the Israelitisches Blinden-Institut only 17 per cent. were found to have speech defects, there being not a single stutterer in the group. When a larger number were given the tests, in the largest school for the blind in Vienna, in which the children represented a mixture of nationalities, 33 per cent. were found to have speech defects. The smaller number having such defects in the Jewish school reduced the total to 28 per cent. ; but it seems significant that in the larger school about one-third of the children of school age had speech defects. This is a higher percentage than we find in the public schools, for non-handicapped children, and compares with the findings in this country in schools for the blind, although in the Vienna schools we found one-third, rather than one-half of the children having speech defects. Even so, it shows that there are more children with speech defects in such schools for handicapped children than we find among children of the same age and grade in public schools for the seeing, and it indicates that remedial work might well be done in these foreign schools also. So far as we were able to ascertain, no such remedial speech-corrective work is provided for in any of the schools for the blind abroad, with the exception of schools where blind-deaf children are educated, and where the manual alphabet is used for speech education. Visual and auditory methods cannot be used with such children, unless there is some remnant of vision or audition, depending upon the severity of the handicap, the age of onset of blindness or deafness, or both, and the native intelligence of the child, as well as the age at which formal education was begun.

The London County Council has established a new

school for the deaf in the outskirts of London, where
there are several blind-deaf children receiving education,
and with these children the manual tactual-cutaneous
method is employed to build up the kinæsthetic imagery,
and to enable the child to form, through the remaining
sensory avenues, such serviceable impressions as may
enable him to associate the knowledge gained in reading
Braille writing, through the fingers, with the corresponding
muscle movements of throat, mouth and larynx to produce
the desired speech sounds. In the same way impressions
between objects touched, surface outlines and configurations built up through touch and through muscle,
joint, and tendon sensations must be linked with corresponding symbols for which images are being built
up by means of Braille reading and by articulate
speech.

Many investigators reporting on surveys of school
children have stated that among Jewish children speech
defect, and particularly stuttering, is more common than in
children of other nationalities. Our findings are just the
opposite of this. Although all children of school age
were examined we did not find a single case of stuttering
in this school. This may be due to early separation from
the home, and to more favourable surroundings than
would be found in the home from which these blind
children come. In the larger school for the blind, however,
among children of different nationalities, 3 cases of
stuttering were found. Of the total number of children
examined in both schools (102), the 3 with stuttering
habits gives a percentage of 2·9. This is a much higher
percentage than that reported by Wallin, Blanton,
Conradi, and others who have given speech surveys
largely by the questionnaire method, depending upon
the teacher's identification of the speech defects, rather
than upon individual tests. It is also somewhat larger
than the figures for the White House Conference Survey
of 1930, as reported by West, Travis, and Camp.[1]

Results of speech tests as given in two schools for the

[1] *The Handicapped Child*, White House Conference Reports, 1931.

blind in Vienna, Austria, to 102 subjects in the Blinden-Erzihungs-Institut and the Israelitisches Blinden-Institut, 1932, follow.

CLASSIFICATION OF SPEECH DEFECTS AFTER
FRÖSCHELS' TERMINOLOGY

|  | Boys | Girls | Total | Per cent. of Group |
|---|---|---|---|---|
| Lateral lisp    .    .    .    . | 3 | 3 | 6 | 20 |
| Multiple interdentality   .    . | 2 | 4 | 6 | 20 |
| Sigmatism    .    .    .    . | 5 | 1 | 6 | 20 |
| Rhinolalia    .    .    .    . | 2 | 1 | 3 | 10 |
| Stuttering    .    .    .    . | 3 | — | 3 | 10 |
| Cleft-palate speech    .    . | 1 | — | 1 | 4 |
| Vocal defect .    .    .    . | 1 | — | 1 | 4 |
| Oral inaccuracy    .    .    . | 1 | — | 1 | 4 |
| Deafness with speech defect   . | 1 | — | 1 | 4 |
| Associative asphasia    .    . | 1 | — | 1 | 4 |
| Total    .    . | 20 | 9 | 29 | 100 |

*Summary*

Of the 102 cases examined, which included all available children of school age, in the two schools, there were 29 cases of speech disorders, or 28 per cent. of the total number.   This was in a ratio of two boys to one girl.

The boys led in the number of cases of sigmatism, stuttering, associative aphasia, rhinolalia, cleft-palate speech, oral inaccuracy, vocal defect, deafness and speech defects as a whole.   The girls led in multiple interdentality. There was an equal number of lateral lispers in both groups of boys and girls.

In conclusion, let us stress the importance of the removal of remedial speech handicaps in blind children, because of their possible bearing upon personality development, happiness and success in making normal social and economic adjustments in those fields which might be open to them, had they merely a defect of vision, but no speech handicap.

# CHAPTER V

## PATHOLOGICAL CONDITIONS AFFECTING THE SPEECH FUNCTION

### DYSARTHRIA IN DISEASES OF THE CENTRAL NERVOUS SYSTEM AND IN NEUROMUSCULAR INVOLVEMENTS

*Conditions and Causes ; Speech Symptoms ; Prognosis*

PATHOLOGICAL conditions affecting the speech function can only be adequately recognized, diagnosed and treated by medical authorities. In many diseases, especially those involving the central nervous system, or the neuromuscular mechanism, one of the early diagnostic signs for the trained clinician is the deterioration of speech. The symptom may range from a comparatively mild disorder with excessive volubility and speech pressure, to a serious impediment, depending upon the degree of cerebropathica, or cerebral involvement present. Sometimes these cases are first referred to the speech pathologist. The layman, parent, or school teacher is often unable to recognize the speech handicap as a symptom of a serious physical disorder, and may refer the child to a speech specialist. For this reason it is exceedingly important that all workers in the speech pathology field should be trained in the minimum essentials of the pathology of speech, diseases in which speech disorders occur, conditions and causes of the handicap, speech symptoms present, and prognosis, with some suggestions as to treatment.

The well-trained speech pathologist or laliatrist should be trained in much the same way as the psychiatric social service worker is trained, that is, should specialize sufficiently in fields tangent to speech so that she may work with the physician, school nurse, psychiatrist, teacher, and parent, to provide the clinical facilities necessary for the removal of a speech handicap.

The growth and development of preventive medicine assumes a greater knowledge on the part of the layman than has been required in the past, and with increasing pressure in the population centres of America ; we are already in the position where we demand more thorough scientific training in our speech-correction specialists than was formerly found necessary.

The author summarizes in this chapter only those types of speech disorders which appear in speech clinics with some frequency, in the public school or college class-room, in centres where medical speech clinics are established, or where child guidance work includes speech correction facilities. We believe that a summary of pathological conditions affecting the speech function will be useful to the teacher and parent as well as to the clinician, because we have found that children referred for speech correction, in the habit clinics of Massachusetts and in child guidance clinics in other parts of the United States constitute a considerable number of the cases referred. In the Holyoke Child Guidance Clinic and in the Northampton Clinic started in 1931, the author has found that the number of children referred for speech defects outnumbered all other types in a ratio of at least two to one. In the Springfield Child Guidance Clinic (1928-9) about one case in seven, referred for mental tests, was a non-reader child. About one child in five had a speech defect, upon the removal of which his social readjustment was partially dependent.

In connection with the Nursery School for the Holyoke Home Information Centre, during two years of psychological testing of " normal children ", the author found cases of children with delayed speech, lisping, letter substitution and stuttering. None of these had been previously recognized as in need of remedial speech training. The discovery of the need of medical and psychiatric advice for these children led to activity on the part of the Director of the Home Information Centre to secure the establishment of a local child guidance clinic.

Many teachers in the field of speech science and various clinicians are genuinely interested in gaining some insight into the causes and conditions under which certain speech disorders occur. The author offers the classification and summaries of certain types of diseases of the nervous system with which speech disorders are associated, in the hope that it may aid the clinical worker in recognizing some important symptoms and in knowing when the child should be referred to the school physician or to a psychiatrist, and that she may also know something of the nature of the disorder, after the medical diagnosis has been given.

Speech defects are by no means invariably found in all of the diseases mentioned. They may be present in a mild form or may be very severe. They may be remedial or they may present a poor prognosis. It is sometimes impossible for physician or speech teacher to predict the effect of remedial speech training, because of the personal element, the intelligence of the child, the nature of his response to remedial measures, his personality, home co-operation and other factors.

We may well bear in mind the psychology of the handicapped child, in discussing speech disorders in such cases, as there seem to be two distinct types[1] and the difference is important in undertaking any form of remedial work. First, there is the child with a moderate handicap, who is willing to be waited upon, often badly spoiled, and willing to remain dependent. Second, there is the child with a serious handicap who will always be a special problem, but whose attitude is that of co-operation, eagerness to improve, and desire to make the best of things. The second child is often the more promising of the two, from the standpoint of remedial results in speech, just as he is more adaptable in other reactions, up to the extent of his special limitations.

[1] Hat, Dr. R. N., *Unpublished Lectures*, Springfield Shriners' Hospital, Mass.

In discussing Dysarthria and the conditions under which it occurs, the author follows the detailed, unpublished classification prepared for the American Society for the Study of Disorders of Speech.[1]

Dysarthria is defined as a speech disorder due to innervation disturbances of articulation associated with trauma, inflammation, degeneration or agenesis of the brain or of the peripheral nerves. The patient's mental processes may remain normal, he may express himself fluently in writing and understand everything he hears and sees, and yet have a speech defect. To those defects which are due to lesions of the central nervous system we shall apply the term Dysarthria Cerebropathica. To those which are due to peripheral nerve lesions or to neuromuscular disorders affecting the speech function we shall apply the term Dysarthria Neuromusculo-pathica.

The speech signs which are roughly characteristic of many of these disorders may be described as follows :—

*A*. ANARTHRIA.—Inarticulateness.
*B*. BRADYARTHRIA.—Laboured Speech.
*C*. MOGIARTHRIA.—Ataxic Speech ; Scanning ; Staccato Speech ; Spastic Speech.

Dysarthria may be caused by lesions in the Pons Varolii, Medulla Oblongata, the supra-bulbar region of the brain, or in the spinal cord. Articulation is sometimes slow and spastic and is generally blurred or indistinct. Dysarthria is one of the characteristic signs in such diseases as pseudo-bulbar palsy, general paresis, cerebral diplegia and disseminated sclerosis, and in various other diseases of the nervous system. The following are some of the more common diseases in which dysarthria occurs, and we present them here in the order in which they will be discussed in this chapter.

[1] Robbins–Stinchfield, *Dictionary of Terms dealing with Disorders of Speech*, 1931.

## I. DYSARTHRIA CEREBROPATHICA

Birth Palsy; Cerebral Palsy of Childhood; Little's Disease; Diplegia; Monoplegia; Hemiplegia; Quadriplegia; Tetraplegia.

Brain Abscess.

Brain Tumour.

Bulbar Paralysis.

Cerebellar Disease.

Cerebral Paralysis; Cerebral trauma or injury; Cerebral arterial disease.

Chorea Minor; Sydenham's Disease.

Chorea Major; Huntington's Disease.

Encephalitis.

Epidemic Cerebrospinal Meningitis.

Epilepsy.

Friedrich's Ataxia; Hereditary Ataxia; Marie's Ataxia.

General Paresis:

    (*a*) Adult form;

    (*b*) Juvenile form.

Hughlings-Jackson Syndrome.

Infantile Convulsions.

Infantile Paralysis; Anterior Poliomyelitis.

Mental Deficiency.

Paralysis Agitans; Parkinson's Disease; Shaking Palsy.

Progressive Spinal Muscular Atrophy.

Spastic Paralysis (see Birth Palsy).

Sclerosis:

    (*a*) Amytrophic;

    (*b*) Disseminated Lateral; Multiple; Insular.

Wilson's Disease; Progressive Lenticular Degeneration.


## II. DYSARTHRIA NEUROMUSCULOPATHICA

Facial or Seventh Nerve Injury or Involvement.

Trifacial or Fifth Nerve Injury or Involvement.

Hypoglossal or Twelfth Nerve Injury or Involvement.

Vagus or Tenth Nerve Injury or Involvement.

F

Acoustic or Eighth Nerve Injury or Involvement.
Glossopharyngeal or Ninth Nerve Injury or Involvement.
Multiple Neuritis ; Polyneuritis.
Myasthenia Gravis ; Vocal Myasthenia.
Miscellaneous ; Laryngismus Stridulus ; Aphonia Spastica.

## I. Discussion of Dysarthria Cerebropathica

### Birth Palsy

Synonyms ; Congenital Spastic Paralysis ; Cerebral
Palsy ; Little's Disease.

*Condition and Causes.*—An injury at birth may cause
paralysis in one or more of the limbs.   It often involves
the motor speech mechanism, through injury to the
cerebral cortex and the brachial plexus.   It is sometimes
due to premature birth, to underdevelopment of the
pyramidal tract, to forceps delivery, or to breech pre-
sentation which causes laceration of the cerebrospinal
meninges.   The spasticity causes irregular movements of
the arms and legs, and frequently of the facial muscles.
The fingers are stiff, and move with slow, irregular movements.   It sometimes resembles chorea spastica.

*Speech.*—When there is a partial paralysis of the
laryngeal muscles, it usually affects the speech mechanism.
There may be glossopharyngeal involvement ; the labial
or lingual muscles may be involved.   The speech defect
may be so slight as to be scarcely perceptible ; it may be
jerky, unrhythmic, " spastic " in type, with " breaks " in
the voice and difficult, laboured utterance.   Cases of
word-blindness, word-deafness, and motor aphasia are
sometimes found which seem to be traceable to injury at
birth.   The latter belong in the dysphasia group.

*Prognosis and Treatment.*—With children presenting a
history of birth palsy it is possible to make very definite
progress in the improvement of speech in many cases.
The prognosis depends upon the extent of involvement—
cerebral, peripheral-nerve, or muscular.   As a prophylactic
measure speech training is often an aid in the general
remedial work, as it stimulates physical activity, aids in

the establishment of co-ordinations between various muscle groups involved, both in speech and in other activities, and enlists the interest of the patient more readily than do some of the routine " gymnastic drills " and other formal disciplines.   If the child is limited in intelligence, progress may be very slow, but with good intelligence, plus a fair degree of motor control and co-ordination of the motor speech centres, good results are often obtained.

Present facilities, even in the public schools, are limited chiefly to education in the early grades for these specially handicapped children, who are usually found in the group known as crippled children.[1]   In a few cities there are high-school classes for such children.   Washington, Chicago, and Los Angeles are typical cities offering special classes for crippled children, including speech training. They also provide bus transportation to and from the school building.   It is a rather thrilling and interesting experience to stand outside the building at the end of a school day, and to see the fine co-operative spirit manifest between children, teacher, janitors, and bus drivers, as these children are aided or encouraged to make their way to the vehicle, and to see them start off on the homeward journey, with cheers and animated faces.   There is little to suggest weaklings or handicapped individuals in their attitudes ;   and their independence and courage is in itself a satisfying by-product of the special educational training instituted for them.

### Congenital Spastic Paralysis ; Cerebral Paralysis of Childhood ; Little's Disease

Congenital spastic paralysis and cerebral paralysis or palsy of childhood are synonyms for Birth Palsy.   Little's Disease is the term applied to all forms of cerebral spastic diplegia.

*Condition and Causes.*—Cerebral paralysis may be caused by injury at birth or by infectious disease.   It is

[1] Solenberger, E., U.S. Bureau of Education, *Bulletin*, 1918, 10.

due to intracranial hemorrhage. In such cases the clot is usually pronounced over the motor area ; if over the speech area, the motor speech function becomes involved. In one case the author saw a child suffering from congenital spastic paralysis, in whom the probable location of the clot, or hemorrhage, had so involved the motor areas of the brain that any prolonged or intense manifestation of voluntary effort, as in speaking, reading or other mental activity, also involved other motor areas. There was an overflow of motor energy, therefore, whenever the child attempted to speak or to read orally, and this was manifested by spastic, inco-ordinate accessory movements of the arms, legs and head, even though the child was able to talk intelligibly and intelligently. This suggests that speech activity normally sends impulses to many motor areas supplying the skeletal muscles, although such impulses are usually inhibited or directed into the active channel of speech itself. Watson has shown this in his studies of sub-vocal muscle activity during the process of silent reading.[1]

*Prognosis and Treatment.*—This form of accessory muscular activity also suggests that the function of speech involves a dominance of motor impulses which under certain conditions may overflow into other motor areas, producing manifestations such as inco-ordinate, spastic, muscular contractions. Interaction between the effect of pure motor activity, as in muscle training, and training in the psychic activities as well as motor-speech activities, may be of considerable benefit to the child. Conversely, over-stimulation of bodily muscular groups might tend to affect the speech centre so as to produce inco-ordination and even stuttering.

The speech may range from chaotic, inco-ordinate or spastic utterance to stuttering, mild or severe. The brain tissue often shows degeneration of the cells of the motor areas. The speech is usually late in developing and is often very defective. Its severity is dependent upon the extent and degree of involvement and may vary from

[1] Watson, John B., *Psychology from the Standpoint of the Behaviourist.*

PLATE VII

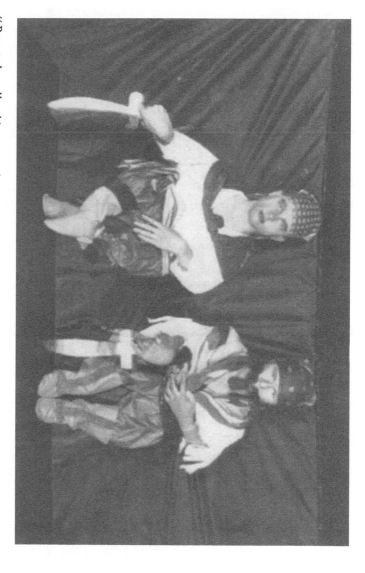

" Puppet shows " and impersonations as an expressional activity for crippled children. Scene from an entertainment at the Orthopaedic Hospital-School, Los Angeles, California. Six children posed to make up this photograph, which illustrates some of the ways in which handicapped children may entertain themselves and others

*(Courtesy of Orthopaedic Hospital, Los Angeles)*

PLATE VIII

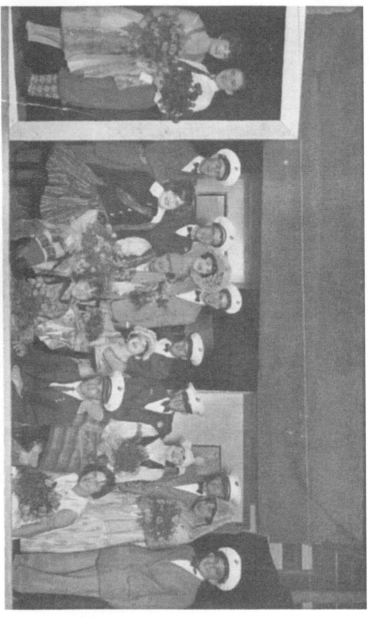

Expressional Activities among Crippled Children. The cast for a play given at the Orthopaedic Hospital-School, Los Angeles
Note the expressive countenances and animation shown

[face p. 85

clumsy utterance to complete disability in controlling the voluntary muscles concerned in speaking. The child may mature physically and yet develop no speech at all. There may be speech, but with marked dysarthria, or with spastic, spasmodic, difficult utterance. The mental retardation may be such that there is little speech aside from idioglossia, lalling and incoherent speech. When the mentality is normal, or only slight retardation is present, speech drill and training is very useful from the standpoint of socialization, physical upbuilding and morale.

### Other Common Forms of Cerebral Palsy

*Monoplegia.*—In monoplegia only a single part is involved. The lesion may be central, or may involve the cerebral, or brachial nerves.

*Diplegia.*—This is a form of paralysis affecting like parts on opposite sides of the body. The form known as infantile diplegia refers to Birth Palsy, which has been already described. Diplegia which appears at birth is known as congenital spastic paraplegia, when it involves the lower limbs and lower part of the body. It affects both motion and sensation and may be of ante-natal, natal or post-natal origin. In the ante-natal form there is an inherent defect in the motor neurons. The condition may be due to pre-natal syphilitic infection. The natal form is due to difficult birth, in which meningeal hemorrhages are common. There are two forms of the post-natal disease, one being chronic and the other acute. In the severe type there may be absence of speech. In milder forms speech is retarded in direct proportion to the degree of brain atrophy or injury.

*Hemiplegia.*—Hemiplegia is paralysis of one side of the body. When it is caused by hemorrhage at birth or during intra-uterine life, it is called Birth Palsy or Infantile Hemiplegia. It may be acquired by infection, or by unusual stress and strain, or traumatic shock. In such cases it is known as an adult hemiplegia. Facial hemiplegia, involving the speech mechanism is not uncommon in speech clinics. The disease may follow cerebrospinal meningitis, convulsions or trauma, with cerebral hemorrhage. It is characterized by paralysis and spasticity, which may be temporary or permanent; and there is usually some mental impairment. It is one of the signs of Little's Disease.[1,2]

*Quadriplegia.*—In this form of paralysis all four limbs are involved. It may be due to birth injury and be classified as a Birth Palsy, or it may be acquired in later life through infection or cerebral hemorrhage.

*Tetraplegia.*—Tetraplegia is a paralysis of all four limbs. It may be the result of injury at birth, as in Birth Palsy, or it may be later acquired, through infection or traumatic shock with cerebral hemorrhage.

*Prognosis.*—In all of the above palsies speech training depends upon the degree of involvement, the extent of the lesion and injury to the parts involved. When the disease is due to a birth injury, speech training may be beneficial, as we have mentioned above. When these lesions are acquired in later life as a result of infection, and the disease is progressive and incurable, the speech deterioration becomes more marked, and speech training is of no benefit.

Dystonia and dysarthria are more severe when the left lenticular nucleus is involved. Aphasia may appear, lasting a month or more. When speech reappears it is scanning and rapid and often is associated with dysphasia. Paralalia literalis may be present, or the inability to utter certain letters. Sometimes the same disorder of speech is present when the right lenticular nucleus is involved. In case the lesion occurs in the medulla oblongata, below the basal ganglia, the cranial nerve facial involvement is on the opposite side of the body. Cerebral softening comes on insidiously, accompanied by headaches, vertigo and swelling, with tingling of the extremities. The softening results from embolism, or thrombosis of the blood-vessels, and may be caused by infectious diseases such as typhoid or diphtheria.[3]

[1] Church-Peterson, *Diseases of the Nervous System*, p. 809.
[2] Mott, F. W., *Arch. of Neurology*, Vol. I.
[3] Nelson, *Living Medicine*, VI, p. 467.

According to Kerley,[1] in Hemiplegia the facial muscles are involved in only a small number of cases. Walking is interfered with and orthopedic surgery or other treatment is frequently necessary. If the third left frontal lobe of a right-handed person is involved, the speech may be aphasic, but is impaired to a lesser degree if the involvement is in the right third frontal lobe. Re-education of the speech function by training the cells in the opposite hemisphere is the common explanation of improvement of speech occurring in such children, under special training.

### Brain Abscess

*Condition and Causes.*—Brain abscesses are generally caused by open scalp wounds or fractures ; they may be a result of purulent inflammation of bone or a bony cavity ; they may come from caries of the bones of the skull by blood-stream infection, following nasal or ear abscesses ; a tuberculous lesion, similarly located, will cause similar symptoms to those of an abscess ; the abscesses may be due to transfer of disease from one area or organ to another. They may be superficial, acute, or subcortical abscesses with a different clinical history in each case. The onset is usually quite sudden, but may remain latent for months or years. There are about four stages in development,—the initial stage ; latent stage ; stage of manifest disease ; and terminal stage. It is before the acute stage has set in that aphasia is often present. It is sometimes associated with alexia. Actual aphasia may not be present, and the speech disorder may be a dysarthria. The speech centres may be affected by pressure from a distance.

*Speech.*—Dysarthria may be present or the speech may be aphasic. Generally the speech is aphasic rather than dysarthric, according to clinical evidence.[2]

*Prognosis.*—Speech training is of value as the abscessed condition begins to clear up, provided the damage is neither extensive nor permanent. When the abscess is

[1] Kerley, *Pediatrics*, p. 568.
[2] Tice, *Practice of Medicine*, IX, p. 615.

active, as just before a rupture, mental dullness is noted. Delirium or hallucinations may be present, due to pressure or absorption of toxins. If rupture takes place through the walls of the lateral ventricles, death rapidly occurs. Abscess may be present in any part of the brain, and it is sometimes found in the frontal lobes or psychomotor areas. Abscess of the left temporal lobe produces sensory aphasia. Abscess in the left frontal lobe in right-handed persons, when the involvement is large, may produce motor aphasia and may involve the right facial nerve. The sensory aphasia and alexia conditions are usually temporary.

### Brain Tumour

*Condition and Causes.* — The majority of all brain tumours are true neoplasms arising from the glioma.[1] The great majority of cases occur before the fiftieth year and sometimes in childhood. They may be either congenital or acquired. Their effect upon the speech depends upon the site involved and whether the motor speech or sensory visual or auditory areas are involved.

*Speech.*—The dysarthria present varies according to the extent of injury, and location of the tumour. In case of frontal lobe brain tumour, motor speech deficiency is usually found with involvement of the left frontal lobe. If the tumour is in Broca's area, there is impairment of vocal expression, and there may be complete motor aphasia, but little if any disturbance of the sensory speech function. Bradyphasia is sometimes found ; also agraphia occurs frequently with tumour of the left frontal lobe. The loss of speech may be temporary, and the motor aphasia be transient. Word deafness and word forgetfulness sometimes are found. As the visual speech centre is in the angular gyrus and supramarginal gyrus of the occipital lobe, word blindness may result from involvement of the angular gyrus in tumours. Dysphasia, in the form of visual aphasia and word blindness or dyslexia results from the involvement of these areas.

---

[1] Cushing, Peter Bent Brigham Hospital, Boston. *Lectures.*

There is difficulty in recalling words and in understanding speech.[1]

*Prognosis.*—The only possible procedure for effecting a cure in this disease is brain surgery, unless there is a gummatous or other infectious tumour. Previous to this, speech training is useless as the tumour is characterized by progressively increasing intracranial pressure. The tumours are more frequent in women than in men and by far the greater proportion appear before the age of forty.

## Bulbar Paralysis

*Condition and Causes.*—In true Bulbar Palsy there is an involvement of the nerves peripheral to the bulbar nuclei. The paralysis starts with the superficial muscles of the tongue ; the tongue becomes atrophied and transverse furrows appear. The muscles used in articulation become involved. As the disease progresses atrophic paralysis takes place involving the palate and vocal cords. The paralysis is due to changes in the motor centres of Pons Varolii and the Medulla Oblongata. It is often associated with enlargement of the thymus gland, when it occurs in childhood. One generally finds a neuropathic heredity in these cases. It is more common in men than in women and occurs about middle age.

*Speech.*—The speech disturbance depends upon the degree of nervous and mental disintegration and upon the muscles involved. Glossolabiolaryngeal paralysis may be present and pronunciation of the gutturals *k* and *g* is impossible. The speech difficulty begins with mispronunciation of dentals and linguals, such sounds as *t, d, j, k, g, l, r* and *s* being difficult. The patient cannot pronounce labials and gutturals, as the disease progresses, and later the speech may become utterly unintelligible. The voice is nasal in the chronic state. The deep reflexes are usually increased, but the intelligence is unimpaired.[2] The patient

---

[1] Bramwell, E., " Diseases of the Nervous System ", *Oxford Medicine*, VI, Part 1.

[2] Tice, IX., *op. cit.*, pp. 289–93.

Osler, *Principles and Practice of Medicine*, p. 931.

is usually short-lived, after the onset of the disease, and speech training can be of only temporary value, as gradual atrophy of the vocal cords causes enfeeblement of the voice.[1]

### Cerebellar Disease—Cerebellar Tumour

*Condition and Causes.*—Tumours of the cerebellum are gliomata [2] and tuberculomata.[3] There is intense pain referred to the occipital region, and it may be accompanied by frontal headache. Nausea and vertigo are almost constant and optic neuritis may be present, with absence of sense of smell. Disturbance of equilibrium and inco-ordination, with a tendency to stagger towards the affected side, is an early and constant symptom. The head is tilted towards the side of the tumour ; nystagmus is also present. The cranial nerves are rarely affected unless the tumour is extra-cerebellar, in which case the acoustic nerve may become involved. Convulsions and tonic spasms are present and the Hughlings-Jackson Syndrome may appear if the tumour is intra-cerebellar. The extra-cerebellar tumours more frequently arise from the acoust'c nerve, and produce more or less deafness, accompanied by tinnitus.[4]

*Speech.*—These tumours may produce unilateral palsies of the fifth, sixth and seventh nerves. The seventh, being the motor facial nerve to muscles of articulation, causes the labial sounds to become affected. Dysarthria is present in this disease when the muscles of articulation are involved. Unilateral facial spasms occur when the facial or seventh nerve is involved. Not only dysarthria, but dysphasia may appear in this disease.[5]

---

[1] Riddoch, G., *Oxford Medicine*, VI, Part 1, p. 303.
[2] Glioma—malignant sarcoma occurring in nerve tissue.
[3] Tuberculomata—tumour caused by the bacillus of tuberculosis.
[4] Tinnitus—ringing of the ears.
[5] *Oxford Medicine*, VI, Part 1, p. 179.

*Cerebral Paralysis ; Cerebral Trauma or Injury ; Cerebral Arterial Disease* (see Birth Palsy and General Paresis)

## Chorea ; St. Vitus' Dance

*Condition and Causes.* — Chorea is characterized by inco-ordinate muscular movements in which the motor control may be partially or wholly lost, and chaotic, irregular muscular activity and twitchings may occur. It occurs more frequently in girls than in boys, and the cause is always some underlying constitutional one. About 50 per cent. of the cases have been associated with rheumatism, according to medical statistics. It is definitely related to tonsillitis and endocarditis. It is of infectious origin and appears to be the result of a vascular degenerative inflammatory encephalitis.

*Speech.*—Unusual speech hesitancy is one of the symptoms of the disease. Awkward muscular movements become apparent, and then irregular and clonic contractions of the muscles occur. When this involves the muscles of the head, face and shoulders, speech disorders occur. Attempts at voluntary control only exaggerate the difficulty.[1]

### Sydenham's Chorea ; Chorea Minor

This form of Chorea is symptomatic of a toxic condition. It is an acute form of the disease, and is also sometimes called St. Vitus' Dance. According to Osler,[2] more than three-fourths of the cases occur between five and fifteen years of age, and in a ratio of one boy to two and a half girls.

*Speech.*—Words are spoken in irregular, jerky fashion, or shot out suddenly, the last syllable being often omitted. According to Glogau,[3] the breathing curve during speech shows choreatic jerkings of the respiratory muscles which cannot be found in other muscles. Swift [4] found a change

[1] Kerley, *op. cit.*, p. 571.   [2] Osler, *Chorea*, 1894.
[3] Glogau, O., *N.Y. Medical Journal*, Jan. 15, 1916, p. 108.
[4] Swift, W. B., *Amer. Journal of Diseases of Children*, Oct. 1914, viii, p. 279.

of voice, most frequently occurring on vowels, less so in whispering, whistling, speaking consonants, air-blowing, and in respiration, the frequency being in the order cited. He speaks of changes in pitch and intensity as one of the symptoms of the disease. A marked change occurs on the Italian *a* (as in arm), and in severe cases the patient may even become mute.

### Huntington's Chorea; Chorea Major

*Condition and Causes.*—Huntington's Chorea is of hereditary, familial origin and usually appears between the ages of thirty and forty. It appears as a dominant trait, and is characterized by choreatic movements, gradual dementia and disturbances of speech. The latter becomes more pronounced as the disease progresses. Speech training is useless as the disease is progressive. The name " St. Vitus' Dance " is sometimes given to this form of chorea, also. The name originates from the fact that during a chorea epidemic, sufferers from the disease sought refuge in St. Vitus' Church in the town where the disease appeared.

Motor symptoms are among the more prominent early signs, and gait, face, and speech are commonly involved. Involuntary muscles may not at first be involved, but later become so, and the reflexes are exaggerated. Facial contortions, thick, drawling speech is heard, with aspirate " *ha* " or " *hem* " sounds, speech being slow and at times impossible. Mental enfeeblement is inevitable. Apraxia is often present.

### Encephalitis; Lethargica

*Condition and Causes.*—In encephalitis there are lesions in the brain, and hemorrhages in the gray matter at the base of the brain. Sometimes the cord is affected. It rarely occurs in children under four years of age and is found in men rather more frequently than in women. Some patients refuse to talk, others develop a slow, monotonous, measured speech. There is a complete change in personality, unstable emotional control, hysterical symptoms, and mental retardation. The onset is usually abrupt. It is easily confused with meningitis. Many cases occurred following the influenza epidemic of 1917–18.[1]

*Speech.*—The dysarthria is more pronounced as the disease progresses. The speech may not be greatly disturbed at first, but there is a progressive deterioration in the speech function, the speech becomes indistinct, blurred and slurring, with mutilation of various syllables. The quality of the voice is also altered as the disease progresses.

*Prognosis.*—Some patients recover. Post-encephalitic treatment for speech improvement may be productive of favourable results, but speech treatment during the course of the disease should not be given. Transfusion has been used with some success in the Children's Division of the Bellevue Hospital (Stetson). With progressive deterioration goes mental impairment, and the speech disturbance usually becomes more marked, therefore.[2]

## *Epidemic Cerebrospinal Meningitis*

*Condition and Causes.* — Cerebrospinal Meningitis is prevalent particularly in childhood and youth, and may be spread by carriers. Cerebrospinal fever is caused by meningococcus germs which enter the system through the mouth or nose. The meninges of the brain are invaded, being extended through the ethmoid and sphenoidal sinuses. If the foramen of Magendie is closed, preventing the spinal fluid from going down into the spinal canal, hydrocephalus may result. Blindness is a frequent result of this disease in infants, unless treated, and deafness is common in adults ; a localized paralysis may occur, according to the motor area of the brain which is involved. Transient facial palsies often occur. The onset is sudden, and the headache is one definite symptom. Disturbed mental condition results and may last far into convalescence or may even become permanent.[3]

---

[1] Church-Peterson, *op. cit.*, pp. 240–41.  [2] Kerley, *op. cit.*, p. 621.
[3] Tice, *op. cit.*, III, pp. 83–103.

*Speech.*—The amount of dysarthria present depends upon the nature and extent of the involvement of brain areas and the degree of mental impairment which results. Exercises of a corrective speech type are usually useful in restoring function, provided invasion by the disease has not been too extensive and the mental impairment has not become permanent.

*Prognosis.*—So far as speech improvement is concerned, the outlook depends upon the degree of involvement of the nervous system and whether there is slight or severe paralysis or other involvement which interferes with the development of normal speech.

## *Epilepsy*

*Condition and Causes.*—It is estimated that 25 per cent. of all mentally deficient children are epileptic.[1] Epilepsy is rare in persons with a good heredity. It involves the highest cortical centres of the brain. With an increase in intracranial pressure comes the epileptic seizure, in which there seem to be five well-marked stages : (1) the aura, (2) loss of consciousness, (3) tonic spasms, (4) clonic spasms, (5) coma or long sleep.

Gowers reports that 50 per cent. of the cases appear between the ages of ten and twenty years and 74 per cent. before the age of twenty. Mental deterioration is progressive in relation to the number of attacks.

*Speech.*—The speech is often thick, the tongue appears heavy, large or unwieldy, the patient speaks as though with mush in the mouth, or with lethargic, lazy speech of the oral-inaccuracy type. Lisping may be present. Patients may show aphasic symptoms or dysarthria, and Oppenheim reports respiratory spasms preceding attacks. Sometimes patients develop delirium, with flight of ideas, rapid speech, motor excitement and hallucinations which lead to violence and crime.[1] The seizures may take the form of unconsciousness or coma due to cerebral anæmia.[2] There is atrophy of the nerve cells and increased reproduction of neuroglia. If the sclerosis and increased glial

[1] Tice, *op. cit.*, IX, p. 434.    [2] Tice, *op. cit.*, pp. 401–14.

tissue is in the region of the speech centres, the speech motor or sensory areas may be involved.

*Prognosis.*—In our experience, speech training is of little value in epileptic cases. It is possible that in State institutions, between attacks, speech training might result in temporary improvement in utterance and be of sufficient value as a prophylactic measure to make it worth while, as patients usually respond to the training. Patients who are under institutional management can profitably receive remedial speech training, but the results are often temporary, as the disease is progressive usually. Cures are rare, but the progress of the disease may be allayed or arrested by some types of treatment.

*Friedrich's Ataxia ; Hereditary Ataxia ; Marie's Ataxia*

*Condition and Causes.*—The onset of Hereditary Ataxia is usually between the fifth and fifteenth years. It is of hereditary origin. According to Kerley [1] it may follow an acute illness. Trembling, jerky movements and inco-ordination accompany the effort to use the extremities, and are apparent in the face when the patient tries to talk or when emotional expression is elicited.[2] Voluntary nystagmus is present and there is a tendency to walk on the outer edges of the feet. Voluntary actions are over-done and the deep reflexes are early lost. The inco-ordination of the extremities is due to the primary degeneration of the dorsal columns and of the spino-cerebellar and pyramidal tracts of the spinal cord. The form which appears before puberty is called " Friedrich's Ataxia ". Marie's Ataxia appears after puberty.

*Speech.*—The speech tends to become " ataxic " or halting. The muscular reactions are delayed and chaotic, with sudden and irregular changes in pitch, alternating with monotony, slow, peculiar and colourless speech. Scanning, staccato speech and ataxic gait are characteristic of Marie's Ataxia, which is the name applied to that form appearing after puberty. There is a dull facial expression, but the mentality may be normal, until late

[1] Kerley, *op. cit.*, p. 600.    [2] Church-Peterson, *op. cit.*, p. 465.

in the course of the disease. Speech disturbances are frequently found.[1] Volume of tone tapers off as in fatigue.

*Prognosis.*— Speech training is of little value in Hereditary Ataxia as the disease is progressive. There may be some temporary benefit to the muscular system as a result of special speech training, but the dysarthria accompanying the advance of the disease becomes more marked, and renders remedial speech work of temporary value.

### *General Paresis*—(a) *Adult form*

*Condition and Causes.*—The symptoms in this disease are so many and varied that it is not within the scope of this work to indicate more than a few of the outstanding features which may be of interest to the teacher in the speech clinic. General Paresis is primarily of syphilitic origin, and tends to attack brain workers or those who are mentally overtaxed. There is a clouding of consciousness, forgetfulness, failing memory, euphoria, unstable emotion, vacillation and obstinacy; the individual is suggestible and often morally irresponsible. Monoplegia, paraplegia and hemiplegia are common and tend to affect the speech function. Complete or partial aphasia may occur, which may be either temporary or permanent.[2]

Paretic dementia, as in general paresis, includes spinal complications and with progress of the disease the dementia becomes more marked.

*Speech.*—The speech is so characteristic that it is easily identified by the physician. It differs in different individuals and may take the form of stuttering, hesitation, scanning, or spasmodic speech, ataxic utterance or other speech disturbance. It sometimes sounds like the speech of the inebriate. Lesions may occur in the motor speech centre of the cortex, or in the bulbar centres which are linked with the motor speech impulses necessary to articulation. Difficulty in enunciation of labial consonants

---

[1] Osler, *op. cit.*, p. 944.    [2] Tice, *op. cit.*, X, pp. 186–91.

is frequent. As the disease progresses the speech may become unintelligible. The speech disturbance is usually, but not always, one of the earliest signs of the disease. Thickness in speech, lisping, difficulty with labials and loss of customary inflections of the voice are characteristic. The handwriting is disturbed and tremor appears. Usually the patient is asked to say such words as "third riding artillery brigade", or "Methodist Episcopal", and in such words the typical speech defect is apparent, as the *r*'s and *l*'s are slurred or dropped by the patient.

The speech is often quite lucid and may exhibit only occasional slips and oral inaccuracies. It resembles the lalling speech of mental deficiency sometimes. Speech deterioration progresses with advance of the disease.

*Prognosis.*—The more serious symptoms of the disease have not been discussed, nor is it within the function of this volume to discuss the far-reaching effects upon the nervous system, of this disease. Speech training is of little value as the disease is progressive and generally incurable. The prognosis is absolutely unfavourable. Arrest may occur, but lapses follow. Mott does not agree with the generally accepted statement "no syphilis, no general paresis",[1] although in the majority of cases the evidence is very strong.

## (b) *Juvenile Paresis*

*Condition and Causes.*—Juvenile Paresis is said to be more common than has formerly been believed. Paretic children are often normal and even brilliant in mental attainment; the onset of the disease is sudden, with mental symptoms, failing memory, and gradual development of a psychosis. The patient alternates between childishness, exaltation and depression, with fears or phobias. The age of onset is from seven to fifteen years after infection. Scars around the mouth, Hutchinson teeth, a history of unfavourable heredity and a positive Wasserman test are the chief diagnostic signs. Epilepti-

[1] Mott, F. W., *Arch. of Neurol.*, I; Church-Peterson, *Diseases of the Nervous System*, p. 809.

G

form and apoplectic attacks occur as in the adult form.[1] Nerve deafness sometimes occurs in children in this disease or in congenital syphilis of the nervous system, and the patient usually becomes totally deaf. If the child has learned to speak normally first, the speech is retained, but it may deteriorate due to the deafness.[2]

*Prognosis.*—If medical treatment for the disease proves favourable, speech training of the type used with aphasics is often fruitful of results. It is assumed that in the case of aphasia involving the left frontal lobe, training may enable one to establish function in the right frontal lobe, compensating for impairment of the opposite side.[3]

### Hughlings-Jackson Syndrome

*Condition and Causes.*—The lesions which are responsible for Hughlings-Jackson Syndrome involve the lowest roots of the Vagus (Tenth) Nerve, the Spinal Accessory and the Hypoglossal nerves. This disease may be due to tumours, organic brain disease or to toxins; to poliomyelitis, syphilis, or to multiple sclerosis. Paralysis of the twelfth nerve causes the base of the tongue to rise on the paralysed side; if the paralysis is bilateral speech is difficult. Hysterical paralysis of the tongue is sometimes reported, but in such cases there is no true degeneration. Cases of hysterical paralysis involving the tongue and speech mechanism have been reported by Tucker.[4]

*Speech.*—The degree of dysarthria present depends upon extent of lesion and progress of the disease. Articulation may be difficult, when the tongue is involved in the paralysis; the movements of the lower jaw may be interfered with by paralysis of the masseteric nerve; paralysis of the facial nerve tends to involve lip movement, and paralysis of the vocal cords may occur through paralysis of the recurrent laryngeal nerve (from Vagus).

[1] Tice, *op. cit.*, X, p. 207.
[2] Mott, F. W., *Oxford Medicine*, " Diseases of the Nervous System," VI, Part 2, pp. 617–22.
[3] Church-Peterson, *op. cit.*, p. 230.
[4] Tice, *op. cit.*, IX, p. 50.

Speech and phonation may be functionally lost in the hysterical form.

*Prognosis.*—The advisability of speech training depends upon the severity of the disease and the prospect of recovery.

### Infantile Convulsions

*Condition and Causes.*—Since a history of infantile convulsions is often found in speech histories of children referred to speech clinics, it is important enough for us to devote space to it here. Convulsions often result from birth injury and may result in serious brain lesions. They sometimes occur previous to the onset of spastic paralysis and may result in idiocy. The cause is insufficient development of the motor centres of the cortex, which discharge too readily. This motor discharge affects the entire muscular structure or any part thereof. Its occurrence indicates cortical irritation. It is sometimes the result of meningitis, tumours, hydrocephalus, or if it occurs in later life, it may result from a blow or severe injury. It has sometimes followed bronchial pneumonia and enterocolitis. In the severe whooping of whooping-cough convulsions sometimes occur due to hemorrhage.

*Speech and Prognosis.*—Speech retardation is often found in these cases because of mental retardation, feeble-mindedness or idiocy. The writer has worked with a case of Aphasia of the auditory-sensory type, the onset of which dates back to the occurrence of convulsions in childhood with resulting septic embolism. There may be a mild dysarthria, or considerable difficulty in articulation, slow cerebration, inadequate motor-speech impulses and a lagging of speech activity. Soon after birth an infant may develop facial grimaces and choreatic twitchings of facial muscles, tendency to stupor and irregular respiration, without true convulsions developing. The prognosis is of course better in such cases than in true convulsions. A history of convulsions with defective mentality, is often found in cases referred for speech treatment, and it is for the physician and teacher to decide to what extent remedial speech training should be given.[1]

### Infantile Paralysis ; Anterior Poliomyelitis

*Condition and Causes.*—Infantile Paralysis is caused by a filterable virus which enters the system through the mouth, nose or throat. The disease has been chiefly studied through the inoculation of monkeys and pigeons, as they are susceptible to the disease. The onset is sudden, with listlessness and loss of appetite, and gastro-intestinal symptoms appear. Regurgitation of food may occur with dull headache or drowsiness. Pains in the extremities occur particularly at night and muscle groups are hypersensitive. Jerky muscular movements occur during rest and tremors may precede the paralysis. Paralysis is not essential to establish the presence of the disease. A non-paralytic form exists, and it is generally conceded that most children have had, at some time, either a mild form of the paralytic, or the non-paralytic form of the disease, and have thus acquired lifelong immunity.[2] In this disease the motor cells in the anterior horns of the spinal cord are involved. This accounts for the loss of motor control which follows.

*Speech.*—The speech often consists of chaotic, jerky utterance ; spasmophemia (stuttering) may be present ; there are often articulatory disturbances such as dysphonia or dysarthria ; the quality and resonance of the voice may be impaired. Speech training is useful in enabling the patient to regain control of the vocal mechanism.

*Prognosis.*—The completeness of recovery and freedom from paralysis of one or more limbs depends upon the severity of the attack. Theoretically one does not expect to find speech disorders associated with this disease, as usually the limbs are involved,[3] through inflammation and destruction of the anterior horn cells of the spinal cord. Since there are sometimes present lesions of the

[1] Kerley, *op. cit.*, p. 533.    [2] Hat, R. N., *op. cit.*
[3] Tice, *op. cit.*, V, p. 335.

subcortical regions of the cerebrum, and also of the basal ganglia and cerebellum,[1] this may account for occasional cases of stuttering which the author has found after an attack of anterior poliomyelitis.

In these cases there was no other disease history to account for the appearance of the speech defect. The speech disturbance takes the form of a subcortical lesion involving the association fibres.

### Mental Deficiency

*Condition and Causes.*—Mental deficiency is not a disease, but rather the result of disease, injury, or of arrested mental development. It may be either hereditary, congenital or acquired. According to the Act of the General Assembly, No. 414, Commonwealth of Pennsylvania, a " mental defective " is defined as a person not mentally ill, but whose mental development is retarded so that he lacks the self-control, judgment, and discretion necessary to manage himself and his affairs, and for whose welfare or that of others, supervision, control or guidance are required. The term includes " idiot ", " imbecile " and " moron ". There are three grades of mental deficiency ; the idiot is one with a mental age below two years ; the imbecile is one with a mental age of two to seven years ; the moron is one with a mental age of seven to twelve years. It is very difficult to distinguish a mentally deficient child from a normal one in the early years, while he is still under three years of age chronologically, but as he advances chronologically, without a corresponding mental development, the discrepancy becomes more apparent.

The subnormal child and the moron may be trained to respond by habit-pattern reactions in many situations and forms of social activity. Through repetition they may be trained in the automaticity of desirable habits and rendered very useful to society as well as more or less self-dependent. Many of the feeble-minded may be

[1] Tice, *op. cit.*, V, pp. 343–359.

satisfactorily trained to do useful types of work and even to become economically self-supporting.  Opportunity classes in the public schools offer adequate educational facilities for a large number of retarded and dull-normal children who can be better trained in the school system than in the home or in a State institution, as they may not be sufficiently handicapped on the mental side to be placed with the mentally deficient in the State schools. Training includes domestic service, caféteria work, commercial work of a mechanical nature, household arts, manual training, vocational activities of various types, sewing and even such work in arts and crafts as are not too difficult for them to understand. [1]

From the educational point of view, the mentally deficient child is one who is two or more years retarded in school progress.  Such children may now be educated without being certified as mental defectives, or as any other type of defective, in fact, both in the United States and in England.  State institutions are so overcrowded that there is an increasing tendency for the public schools to take over the education of mentally deficient children, whenever this is feasible. [2]

*Speech.*—Tredgold [3] finds that a great many cases of word-blindness and word-deafness occur in dull or retarded children.  Word-blindness or alexia concerns only written or printed words.  The child says the alphabet, recites and spells, but can't read by sight or recognize the letters of the alphabet.  He therefore has difficulty in learning to read and write.  In some, the inability also includes figures as well as letters.  The difficulty is probably due to slow or defective development of certain cells of the brain.  Tredgold finds that about 1 in 2000 school children are word-blind. [3]  In mental defectives word-blindness occurs in 1 in 20 children and is four times commoner in boys than in girls.

[1] Church-Peterson, *op. cit.*, p. 851.
[2] Tredgold, *Mental Deficiency*, 1914.
[3] Tredgold, *Unpublished Lectures*, Central Association for Mental Welfare, London, 1931.

Word-deafness, according to Tredgold, is due to congenital auditory imperception. Such children are not deaf in the ordinary sense, as they can hear, but their sound perception is not up to the normal. Many such children are dull, and develop a speech defect such as idioglossia or lalling. Such children often have difficulty in spelling, and in writing from dictation.

*Prognosis.*—In the past the advisability of speech education and correction for mentally deficient children has been much questioned. There is the danger that such children may be exploited by unscrupulous teachers, without great speech improvement being obtained. " Guarantees " of the attainment of normal speech have even been given to over-credulous parents by such " teachers ". The author feels convinced from her experience with mentally deficient children both within and without the State institutions, that many of them, particularly those of the moron or dull-normal level, could profit by speech correction work, rightly given.

We have already called attention to the fact that schools for the blind, deaf and crippled children stress the importance of removing every remedial handicap from children who already possess some special drawback. We believe that to this list should be added the mentally deficient child who is sufficiently bright to profit by remedial speech training which would make him a more useful member of society, since he is frequently released from the institution, or else never reaches the same, and is placed in positions where some responsibility is placed upon him, and in which he could save both time and money to his employers, were his speech more acceptable and easier to understand. One has only to pass through any average American city as a tourist, and stop for the usual services in stores and garages, or upon street-cars, to hear any number of " speech defects " in the civilian population. Not all of them are due to defective mentality, of course, but there is no doubt a larger number of dull-normal or retarded adults in our civilian population, among whom speech defects are the rule, than we commonly realize.

To be more specific, we believe that every State institution and every school where there are opportunity classes for the dull-normal, should employ a teacher of speech correction for such children as are able to profit by such instruction. Through many of the ordinary kindergarten activities and through music, rhythmic games, singing, nursery rhymes, poems, object-training, pictures and reading, a fine service can be performed which will improve the speech as well as general perceptual ability. Development of the auditory and motor as well as of the visual speech centres should come first. Tongue, lip and mouth gymnastics to counts or music may train in rhythm and muscular responses. Lip imitation of sounds may be used in case of .deafness. One usually proceeds from the teaching of simple sounds, such as the labials, with vowels, as in *mama, pa-pa, ba-ba,* to linguals *t, d* and *n,* applying them to other words containing these sounds, and so on through the entire list of consonant and vowel sounds.[1]

### *Paralysis Agitans ; Shaking Palsy ; Parkinson's Disease*

*Condition and Causes.*—Paralysis agitans is a sclerotic process of the posterior and lateral columns of the spinal cord, with sclerotic areas in the corpus callosum and the anterior commissures. It is primarily a disease of old age or of alcoholism, but there is also a juvenile form. Some authorities state that most of the cases occur in persons between twenty and thirty years of age. The disease is progressive and the basal ganglia are involved. Persistent muscular exercise is sometimes fruitful of good results, and for this reason speech training may be of temporary benefit, especially during periods of remission. The disease occurs twice as often in men as in women.

*Speech.*—The speech is deliberate, dull, monotonous, slow, and spastic. It may be characterized by hurried enunciation or by abrupt termination. Monosyllabic

[1] Stinchfield, S. M., *Speech Pathology*, " Vowel-Consonant Chart," p. 141.

speech is frequent. There is no halting, as in Friedrich's ataxia. Laryngoscopic examination usually reveals tremor and sometimes rigidity of the vocal cords. As already stated, speech training is of temporary benefit only, as the disease is progressive.[1]

## Progressive Muscular Atrophy

*Condition and Causes.*—In this disease there is progressive degeneration of the motor nucleii in the medulla and pons, especially in the nucleii of the hypoglossal and facial nerves and also of the ninth, tenth and eleventh cranial nerves. Occasionally the motor fibres of the fifth nerve are involved. It affects the muscles of the tongue, of mastication and of the pharynx and larynx. Chvostek believes that there is also a disturbance of the parathyroids in this disease. Changes in the spinal cord resemble those of amyotrophic lateral sclerosis. Injuries to the head at birth may cause a tumour-like swelling, due to the tearing of the brain covering. Two types are mentioned in the literature, the bulbar type and the spinal type.

*Bulbar Type.*—In Progressive Bulbar Paralysis (Bulbar Palsy) fibrillary twitchings occur, locally, and the speech may be more or less involved with progress of the disease. It is found occasionally in children, but more often in advanced stages of amyotrophic lateral sclerosis or ophthalmoplegia.[2]

*Spinal Type.*—In Progressive Spinal Muscular Atrophy of the spastic type, there is wasting of the musculature, especially of the upper extremities, and some tonic paralysis. The reflexes tend to become exaggerated and speech is affected when the lips, tongue or larynx are involved. The onset is gradual and the disease is progressive.

*Speech.*—Dysarthria appears first and is followed by difficulties in swallowing, in phonation and in respiration.

---

[1] Church-Peterson, *op. cit.*, p. 572 ; Wilson, S. A. R., *Oxford Medicine*, VI, Part I, p. 288.

[2] Collier, *Oxford Medicine*, VI, Part I, p. 330.

Consonants become less distinct and finally are inaudible. Nasality is present due to the inactivity of the soft palate. The dysarthria may vary from mild to severe, but speech involvement is more marked as the disease progresses.

*Prognosis.*—Treatment is chiefly palliative. Electric treatments give beneficial results. The value of speech training is doubtful as the disease is progressive and there is a labioglossopharyngeal involvement. In the progressive bulbar type death usually results in from one to seven years after the onset of the disease. As this disease progresses the patient is unable to divide words into syllables and they are drawn out into one long inarticulate, monotonous sound. The speech defect is apparent early in the course of the disease, which begins with the distal ends of the limbs and with tongue, lips, palate and larynx. The movements are rhythmic oscillations of the flexor and extensor muscles, characterized by slowness of movements and gait.

## Spastic Paralysis

This has been discussed under the heading Birth Palsy.

## Sclerosis

### A. *Amyotrophic Lateral Sclerosis*

*Condition and Causes.*[1]—The etiology of Amyotrophic Lateral Sclerosis is unknown, although there is found to be present a weakness of the entire nervous system. The onset is usually between the ages of twenty and thirty-five years. It comes on gradually, with muscular weakness, atrophy and rigidity, beginning in the hands but involving the glossolabial region in the third stage, causing paralysis, with slow, monotonous speech ; the lips begin to atrophy, and there is wasting of the muscles of the larynx and lower face. Talking and whistling may be impossible, and muscles of respiration are often involved so that the patient may die of respiratory difficulty.

---

[1] Tice, *op. cit.*, IX, pp. 308, 317.

The disease affects the lateral columns and the anterior grey matter of the spinal cord.

*Prognosis.*—From the standpoint of training, there is no purpose in speech drill, as the disease is progressive and incurable. The increasing stiffness of the tongue, immobility in facial expression and fatigue in attempting to talk, render such work increasingly difficult and without satisfactory results.

### B. *Multiple Sclerosis ; Disseminated Lateral Sclerosis ; Insular Sclerosis*

*Condition and Causes.*—Volitional tremor, scanning speech and nystagmus are characteristic of this disease. It is more common in women than in men and may attack several members of the same family. It usually appears between the ages of twenty and forty. Scattered patches of sclerosis are found throughout the brain and spinal cord. Its cause is unknown, although constitutional anomalies are believed to be the cause. The patient is predisposed by reason of defective heredity and defective nervous tissue. The disease may appear at about the age of puberty, when the nervous system is unstable. Sensation is unaffected. The onset is gradual and there is speech impairment of the dysarthria type, which increases as the disease progresses. Tremor is often present. The disease is sometimes mistaken for hysteria.

*Speech.*—Scanning speech is present and the mental symptoms are variable and often uncontrollable. As the disease progresses there is a slow pronunciation of words, and the speech becomes more and more halting, colourless and unemotional. In addition to the characteristic scanning, the patient divides words, makes long pauses, and utters monotonous, rhythmical, cadent tones, as in scanning Latin poetry.[1] Sometimes the speech is staccato or syllabic in utterance.[2] The speech defect is probably

[1] Scripture, E. W., Records of Speech in Disseminated Sclerosis, *Brain*, 1916, xxxix, p. 455.

[2] Stewart, T. Grainger, *Oxford Medicine*, Part 2, p. 625 ; Osler, W., *Principles and Practice of Medicine*, p. 952.

due to cerebellar disturbance in this disease. It ranges from anarthria or aphonia, to dysarthria and dysphonia. As the disease is progressive and recovery rare, speech training is of little value.

### Wilson's Disease

*Condition and Causes.*—Wilson's Disease involves the softening and degeneration of the lenticular nucleus without any involvement of the internal capsule. There is often spasmodic, jerky muscular action, the speech organs being affected according to the degree of hypertonicity and lack of voluntary control.

It may attack more than one member of the family, although it is not a hereditary disease. It is progressive and usually fatal, the duration being from a few months to five to seven years. It is characterized by bilateral, involuntary movements of the extremities and sometimes of the head and trunk. There is hypertonicity of the skeletal muscles, and the face is set in a " spastic " smile.

*Speech.*—The speech areas may not be involved, but difficulty in articulation may be present, due to the hypertonicity of the muscles of the jaw, lips, tongue and pharynx. Volitional acts become difficult, and therefore the speech may become involved. The motor quality of speech becomes spastic. Dysarthria is a constant symptom. It may degenerate into complete anarthria.[1] As speech is gradually lost there is often a tremor of the vocal cords. Emotional over-reaction is characteristic.[2]

### II. DYSARTHRIA : NEUROMUSCULOPATHICA

#### Facial or Seventh Nerve Injury ; Facial Paralysis

*Condition and Causes.*—Facial paralysis is characterized by paralysis of the seventh cranial or facial nerve, and is

[1] Inability to enunciate intelligibly a single word or syllable.
[2] Wilson, S. A. R., *op. cit.*, pp. 264–68.

often due to pressure from forceps at birth. It may be due to trauma following surgery, to severe exposure, to toxic conditions, to cerebellar disease, or to rheumatism.[1] Dysfunction of the seventh nerve may be due to central or peripheral disease or injury. In Bell's Palsy, a form of this disease, there is neither voluntary or emotional movement of the facial muscles. A " tic " of facial muscles is sometimes present. The facial is the great motor nerve supplying the muscles of expression. One branch, the chorda tympani, carries taste sensation from the anterior two-thirds of the tongue. The seventh nerve may be irritated by intracranial tumours, tubercles, gummata, abscess or hemorrhage. Some irritation, from pressure, may arise, in the parotid gland through which it passes. If the injury or pressure is sufficient to cause paralysis, the facial muscles of the side which is paralysed are more involved in the lower part of the face, as the upper facial muscles receive some bilateral innervation. In case of hemorrhage in the internal capsule or upper portion of the pons a hemiplegia will result with facial involvement of the same side ; but if the lesion is in the middle or lower part of the pons, the facial involvement will be on the side opposite from the hemiplegia. Temporary paralysis, as in Bell's Palsy clears up ; the permanent types are more often the result of a central lesion, tumour, trauma, or of unskilled mastoid operation ; and the prognosis in these cases is less favourable.

*Speech.*—The speech disorder or dysarthria present depends upon the extent to which the nerve is involved, and the articulatory muscles concerned.

There is sometimes a compensatory reaction of the muscles of the opposite side of the face, so that speech training aids in muscular control of the injured side, and speech improvement may be secured after considerable practice and persistence. The prognosis is more hopeful when the cause is other than brain disease.

[1] Kerley, *op. cit.*, p. 597.

## Fifth Nerve or Trifacial

*Condition and Causes.*—The fifth nerve supplies the pterygoids, temporal, masseter, and mylohyoid muscles. The lingual branch of the inferior division supplies the anterior two-thirds of the tongue, carrying sensation. This nerve has both sensory and motor functions, supplying most of the head and face, superficially. Lesions of that part of the motor area of the cortex which is associated with this nerve, will produce spasms or paralysis, according to the nature of the lesion. Multiple sclerosis and tabes are given as causes of involvement of the nucleus of the fifth nerve.[1] Among motor symptoms are paralysis of the mandibular muscles controlling the jaw. Facial hemiatrophy may follow diseases of the fifth nerve. Neuritis and neuralgic pains are often traced to disease of this nerve or to irritation of some of its branches.

*Speech.*—Inability to control the jaw, when this occurs in injury to the fifth nerve or in disease, affects the speech. Nerve irritation and neuritis might be sufficient to induce stuttering in children or adults, under stress or strain, following injury or disease to this nerve. Other types of speech disturbance of the dysarthritic type depend upon nature and extent of involvement.

*Prognosis.*—Treatment to restore the nerve to its normal condition is recommended, rather than speech training. The prognosis depends upon nature and extent of the lesion, and whether there is central or peripheral nerve involvement.

Inability to control the movements of the jaw affect the speech. Nerve irritation and neuritis arising from this condition might be sufficient to produce stuttering in a child or adult, under certain conditions of stress and strain.

## Hypoglossal or Twelfth Nerve Injury

*Condition and Causes.*—The Hypoglossal Nerve is the motor nerve for the muscles of the tongue. This nerve

---

[1] Church-Peterson, *op. cit.*, p. 117.

may be injured or diseased anywhere in the pathway from the cortex to the peripheral branches, producing spasm, paresis or paralysis, according to the extent of involvement. Speech difficulties are partly due to lingual spasms when this nerve is involved. Over use or fatigue may produce a condition known as aphthongia, which is not unlike writer's cramps. Widespread cortical lesions in the motor tract also produce a one-sided paresis or paralysis of the tongue. The tongue deviates towards the non-paralysed side, whether the lesion is peripheral or central. In this condition tongue atrophy follows. In the bilateral type of disease the speech disorder is very severe, as nearly all the consonants are slurred, due to the inability to control the tongue.[1]

*Prognosis.*—This depends upon the severity of the lesion, extent of involvement, and degree to which the nerve is injured or diseased, and other possible complications such as muscle spasms. Compensatory movements of the uninvolved opposite side of the tongue often enable the patient to improve his articulation, following involvement of this nerve, and for this reason speech exercises are often valuable.

### Vagus or Tenth Nerve Injury

*Condition and Causes.*—The superior laryngeal branch of the Vagus controls the epiglottis and the vocal cords through the cricothyroid muscle. The recurrent laryngeal nerve, another branch of Vagus, supplies sensation to the trachea and larynx, below the vocal cords, and controls the remaining intrinsic muscles of the larynx. Paralysis of the superior laryngeal nerve may therefore prevent the tensing of the vocal cords ; paralysis of the recurrent laryngeal nerve may prevent abduction or adduction of the cords. The chief adductors are the lateral crico-arytenoids and transverse arytenoid muscles. It is believed that the lateral, internal slip of the cricothyroid muscle, inserting below the vocal cords, is concerned

[1] Church-Peterson, *op. cit.*, pp. 152–54.

with the production of voice registers, by altering the length of the vibrating portions of the cords.

*Speech.*—Speech disturbances result from paresis of either of the above-named nerves. In case the superior laryngeal nerve is involved, there is inability to produce tension of the cords, and the voice is low and unsteady. A hoarseness may result from involvement of the recurrent laryngeal nerve causing disturbed contractions of the thyroarytenoid muscles which parallel the cords. Unless these muscles contract with absolute accuracy, the vibrations of the cords are altered and a mixture of sounds will result. Also, volume of voice is impaired by weakness of the adductor muscles, preventing sufficient approximation of the cords. A complete loss of voice or aphonia, may result from hysterical paralysis of the adductors. Laryngeal spasms are not uncommon, but the attacks are of short duration. Spasmodic " nervous coughs " are described by Church and Peterson.[1] The neurasthenic person is more liable to attacks of laryngeal spasms and hysterical seizures, including mutism, than is the more stable individual.

*Prognosis.*—This depends upon the nature of the involvement. If a functional neurosis is present, the outlook is favourable, as in hysterical mutism. If an inflammatory condition involves the nerve supply or the muscles themselves, complete recovery is to be expected, unless permanent damage has resulted from the inflammatory processes as might be expected in some cases of central nerve lesions, as in tumours of the medulla oblongata or some infectious disease which produces destruction of nerve tissue. Tuberculosis of the larynx may produce destruction of both the musculature and membranes in the region of the cords. When the extent of the injury has been discovered and treatment prescribed, voice exercises should be given only under the direction of a physician. Treatment depends upon the nature of the disturbance and the extent of injury, disease or dysfunction.

---

[1] Church-Peterson, *op. cit.*, pp. 139–48.

## Acoustic or Eighth Nerve

One branch of the eighth nerve supplies the vestibular portion of the inner ear, and another branch supplies the cochlear division of the same. Hysterical deafness is often mistaken for eighth nerve injury, but is usually a transient condition which renders the patient unable to hear temporarily. Although the deafness disappears, the patient often has relaxed auditory attention and habit of listening, so that he remains apparently deaf. Lip-reading in such cases only tends to prolong the difficulty. Cortical deafness following concussions or lesions in the cortical centres are rare. Transitory deafness with auditory amnesia are a part of a condition in which other senses participate.

## Glossopharyngeal or Ninth Nerve

The Ninth or Glossopharyngeal Nerve supplies the posterior one-third of the tongue and the epiglottis. It sends branches also to the superior constrictor muscle, the soft palate, pillars of the fauces and parotid gland. Lesion of this nerve results in anæsthesia of the pharynx and loss of sensation in the back of the tongue. Lesions of the ninth, tenth and eleventh nerves cause palsy of the palate, pharynx and larynx in varying degrees.

There are many other diseases involving the nervous system and peripheral nerve supply, but we have presented here only those in which we find disturbances of speech sufficiently serious to cause the patient to be referred rather frequently to a speech pathologist or speech clinical worker.

## Multiple Neuritis ; Polyneuritis ; Beri-Beri

*Condition and Causes.*—Multiple neuritis is primarily a disease of adult life, but may occur in childhood. It begins in the extremities of the body. There is a degeneration of the nerve trunks, and the spinal cord is often involved. Lesions in the brain and cerebellum have

H

also been found. The highest nerve centres are frequently involved. There are sensory disturbances and mental symptoms, and the nerve trunks are very sensitive. A characteristic gait appears, known as " steppage " ; the muscles of the forearm and hands are affected ; muscles of the face and neck when involved, may include the eyes, tongue, throat, and larynx ; also the diaphragmatic, respiratory, and heart muscles are affected. Mental disturbance is quite common in polyneuritis, influencing the temperament and character of the patient unfavourably.

Polyneuritis is primarily a nutritional disturbance in which there is a toxic condition of the organism. Auto-intoxication and infections are common causes.

*Speech.*—Memory is affected by the disease and the patient forgets easily. Repetitious speech is common. Discrepancies in statements are a key to the degree of mental impairment present. Speech training depends upon the severity of the disease and the prognosis. Exercises for the speech musculature are helpful, after the disease has reached its stationary period or has been arrested or cured.

*Prognosis.*—Complete recovery is possible, when the cause of the disease is one which can be removed.

## Myasthenia Gravis

*Condition and Causes.*—According to Osler, this disease belongs to the third decade ; but a chronic form may appear at about the age of puberty. Muscles innervated by bulbar nucleii are first affected. Muscles of mastication, neck, face, and eyes are often involved. It is characterized by weakness and paralysis of musculature. The weakness disappears after rest, but appears earlier each succeeding day as the disease progresses. It appears in women more frequently than in men. It is sometimes held to be of post-encephalitic origin.[1] Tongue, lips, and pharynx may be paralysed.

*Vocal myasthenia* is a form of the above. The basis

[1] Archiner, D. M., *Arch. of Neurol. and Psychia.*, xxiv, 3, pp. 570–73.

for the disease is usually a neuropathic heredity, the muscles being the seat of the disease.

*Speech.*—As the muscles degenerate there is a weakness of the muscles of articulation and disturbances of speech result. The singer may falter at the end of his song from laryngeal muscle fatigue. Soft palate fatigue is present and causes nasality to appear in the voice. Total paralysis of the laryngeal muscles does not take place, but the voice becomes hoarse, low pitched, and the patient cannot shout because of weakness of the intrinsic muscles of the larynx and of the respiratory mechanism. The voice tires easily. Speech is clearer in the morning than in the afternoon, and there is a vocal myasthenia of phonation, although there is no true dysarthria. Archiner found no paralysis of labial, palatal, lingual or pharyngeal muscles in the cases described by him, but the speech was muffled much as though the nostrils were obstructed.

*Prognosis.*—The prognosis for myasthenia gravis is poor, as the patient may die through asphyxia. If the brain stem escapes injury, the patient often recovers. The cause of the disease appears to be somewhat uncertain. No voice treatment should be given until the patient has fully recovered, as extra effort retards recovery.

*Miscellaneous.*—There are other less common forms of dysarthria in nervous diseases, such as laryngismus stridulus, aphonia spastica, Bell's Palsy, and in lesions or injury to the eighth or to the ninth nerve. Spasms of the larynx may be : first, adductor spasms ; second, spasms of the tensors of the vocal cords ; third, a spasmodic laryngeal cough, common in childhood and known as *laryngismus stridulus*.

*Aphonia spastica* appears in a neurosis due to overuse of voice, and causes sudden interruption during speech. Spasmodic laryngeal coughing is often hysterical.[1]

---

[1] *Oxford Medicine*, VI, Part 2, pp. 703-4.

# CHAPTER VI[1]

## DYSPHEMIA, OR BACKGROUNDS WHICH PRODUCE THE STUTTERER

## DYSPHONIA, OR VOICE DEFECTS

DYSPHEMIA is defined as intermittent and variable nervous disorders of speech accompanying certain psychoneuroses. Spasmophemia or stuttering is one of the best-known forms of this type of speech disorder. Spasmophemia is characterized by cramps or spasmodic contractions of the muscles concerned in speech, by spasmophilia or by rapid repetition of a word or its initial letter or syllable, and is usually accompanied by the fear of becoming ridiculous. It may take the form of aphemia or dumbness, of paraphemia or neurotic lisping, of spasmophemia or stuttering (stammering) ; of agitophemia or nervous, agitated speech.

### APHEMIA

Aphemia or dumbness consists of temporary or prolonged abstinence from speech. It sometimes takes the form of hysterical mutism. It was a form of hysterical seizure which was not uncommon during the World War, when sudden fright or panic seized an individual in a dangerous situation. *Aphemia pathematica* is loss of speech due to intense fright or to rage, anger, or strong emotion, which temporarily overpowers the speech impulse. It tends to occur in over-emotional, temperamental individuals, or in uncontrolled, erratic or infantile personalities. Aphemia plastica is voluntary muteness. It ranges from the wilful silence of a stubborn child or adult, to the refusal to talk which is common among psychopathic individuals seen in mental disease hospitals. Aphemia spasmodica or spasmodic dumbness is found in neurotic individuals and is frequently associated with

[1] *See also* Chap. VII., Dyslogia.

a history of disease. It may occur in chorea, or may be associated with stuttering or other speech defect; it may be found in the excessively nervous, over-stimulated child or adult.

## PARAPHEMIA

This is a form of dysphemia characterized by the substitution of a complete interruption of an outgoing breath stream for its more or less delicate constriction as required for such consonants as *f, v, s, z* and *th*, changing *f* to *p*; *v* to *b*; *s* and surd *th* to *t*; *z* and sonant *th* to *d*. It is caused by excessive muscular tension. According to Scripture [1] it is allied to stuttering in its causation, namely fright, nervous strain, or emotional disturbance. It differs from negligent lisping in that it appears in nervous persons rather than in dull, phlegmatic personalities, and the muscular movements are cramplike, instead of careless.

*Treatment.*—All of the disorders in this group should be treated as nervous disturbances. The treatment appropriate to a given individual may call for a readjustment of other persons to the patient, or if this is impossible, it may call for the removal of the patient to a more favourable environment during such time as is necessary for treatment or re-education to overcome the difficulty. Mental and physical hygiene, simplification of school programme, longer hours of rest and sleep, or changes in diet and habits of exercise may be needed. Electro-therapy and hydro-therapy are also useful. The speech training should not be forced upon the child as a necessary evil, but if it can be given as a form of play, or beneficial exercise and the child's co-operation can be secured to enable him to assist the teacher in her therapy, the training may be co-ordinated with other mental and physical therapy under medical direction.

## AGITOPHEMIA

Agitophemia, or tachyphemia is a form of dysphemia characterized by morbid rapidity or volubility of speech

[1] Scripture, E. W., *Stuttering and Lisping*, 1914, p. 185.

in nervous patients. Nervous, excitable men and women are prone to speak in this way. They are apparently unaware of the speech-urge, or speech-pressure and volubility as being responsible for their frequent and excessive fatigue.

## SPASMOPHEMIA

Many synonyms are current to describe various forms of speech hesitation, stuttering or stammering, which we have grouped under spasmophemia. The following are perhaps the more common titles found in speech disorder literature :—

  (*a*) Convulsive hesitation.
  (*b*) Speech blocking.
  (*c*) Speech hesitation.
  (*d*) Logospasm.
  (*e*) Mogilalia.
  (*f*) Spasmodic speech.
  (*g*) Speech stumbling.
      1. Dysarthria literalis—stammering.
      2. Dysarthria syllabaris spasmodica—stuttering.

Spasmophemia is not the most common of speech disorders, but it is probably the best known and most easily identified. It is a greater handicap to the individual than is a lisp or a vocal peculiarity, as it often impairs the power of making a desirable social adjustment, and even destroys the happiness of the individual through its effect upon his social and economic life. Although there are still many problems in connection with the etiology of stuttering which have yet to be solved, I wish to emphasize here that stuttering, with a functional basis, may be cured or at least greatly improved in the majority of cases.

This speech disorder has an ancient history. Early writers mention sudden recoveries which seem to indicate the hysterical nature of some forms of stuttering which were present in ancient times. This is only one of the possible causes however. The World War taught us much about the disturbances of speech. Sometimes complete loss of voice, or aphemia, occurred in connection with an hysterical reaction due to severe fright, or shock. When the speech returned, it often took the form of a severe stutter, at first. This usually became milder as the effect of the seizure wore off, and was sometimes followed by complete recovery of voice and speech. Such factors as excessive fatigue, prolonged anxiety or strain in a person of neurotic temperament played an important part in the etiology.

Varied definitions of stuttering have been given in medical and psychological literature. It has been defined as an " anxiety neurosis ", as " difficult, unrhythmical speech characterized by involvement of the oral mechanism " ; as related to hysteria ; as due to lack of cerebral dominance ; [1] as due to defective auditory or visual imagery ; [2] as traceable to the lack of some important hormone in the blood, or to bio-chemical changes within the organism.[3]

Blanton has found that there seems to be an hereditary basis for stuttering, in that there often is transmitted to offspring a congenital weakness of the nervous system or of the speech organs themselves which sooner or later is manifested in the form of a speech defect. It may be that the child stutters ; it may be that his speech is of the oral-inaccuracy type, with numerous letter-substitutions and mutilations of words, sounds or syllables. With increased effort to speak, more blocking occurs, showing that the speech hesitation or stumbling is not under voluntary control at all times. Spasmophilia following such diseases as latent (infantile) tetany and rickets in childhood, often persist in the form of weakness and flabbiness of the facial musculature of the stutterer. The spasm is not a true one, however, since it may be

---

[1] Travis, L. E., *Speech Pathology*, Ch. V.

[2] Bluemel, C. S., *Stammering and Cognate Defects of Speech*, pp. 91–102.

[3] Kopp, G., *Bio-Chemical Studies of the Cause of Stuttering*, Symposium, Amer. Soc. for the Study of Disorders of Speech, pp. 1–6.

produced voluntarily by the stutterer, as mentioned by Dunlap,[1] and, under certain conditions, such " spasms " may be brought under voluntary control. This is not the case with the true spasm.

Many excitable children, in learning to talk, repeat syllables, words or phrases. If the situation is treated casually, not dramatically, by parents, the child may naturally discard the excessive rapidity or blocking in speech. Imitation at this time easily leads to the establishment of a permanent habit and it is not desirable that children should be associated with other stutterers. The mere effort to compete with other children in the home or on the playground is sufficient to induce stuttering in excitable or neurotic children. If the child becomes excited or irritated over his inability to gain attention as easily as do the older children of the family, he endeavours to gain attention by talking faster, or louder, or by temper display, cluttered speech and the like. This may easily lead to the acquisition of speech-hesitancy. Parents should train such children to talk more slowly, to speak without undue strain or excitement. Over-attention and consciousness of the habit on the part of the stutterer himself, in social situations in which he feels inferior to the adults or older children present, is sufficient to produce a temporary habit of speech hesitation, blocking, " spasmodic " utterance which may easily become set as a part of the habitual speech reactions. The longer it persists, the more difficult it is to permanently overcome.

Orton reports on the heredity nature of stuttering and of left-handedness [2] where there is a neuropathic background. Robbins, in studies made in Massachusetts including stutterers dealt with over a period of several years, finds that among 2000 patients over 50 per cent. had one or more relatives who stuttered.

---

[1] Dunlap, Knight, *Researches*, Johns Hopkins Clinic.

[2] Orton, S. T., " Familial Occurrence of Disorders in Acquisition of Language ", *Eugenics*, Vol. III, 4, Apr. 1930, 8 p.

*Ibid.*, " A Physiological Theory of Reading Disability and Stuttering in Children ", *New Eng. Jour. of Med.*, Nov. 1928, Vol. 199.

Stuttering occurs in many patients having diseases of the central nervous system. Forms of stammering are found in dysphasic patients and in psychotic and mentally deficient individuals. The prognosis in such cases is discouraging, and speech training is rarely worth while. It is sometimes important, however, from the standpoint of mental hygiene. The most promising outlook for overcoming habits of stuttering are found in cases where there is a rather superficial functional, rather than a pathological or organic-disease history.

Histories [1] show that the onset often follows severe fright, traumatic shock, due to injury or to surgical operation, severe illness or childhood disease. Rickets and latent tetany have been mentioned as causative factors. The laryngospasm accompanying tetany in infancy, may easily lead to the establishment of " spasmodic speech " as a permanent feature of the speech habits. [1] " Spasms " of the facial musculature often remain, after tetany has disappeared, and the Chvostek's sign found in true tetany seems to leave a counterpart in a permanent weakness of the facial musculature over the course of the facial nerve. This is found on tapping the side of the face, lightly, as in examination for Chvostek's sign. In true tetany there is a swift, transient contraction of muscles about the mouth or eyes, depending upon the branch of the nerve which has been stimulated. Often a quivering or flabbiness of musculature or a fibrillary twitching of the cheek muscles may be seen, associated with stuttering, and it is possible that there may be a background of latent tetany in such cases as has been suggested.

Rickets and tetany furnish a favourable soil for the development of habits of cluttering and stuttering, as such children often are unduly irritable, excitable and neurotic, even after the childhood disease or illness has disappeared. Stuttering is also found among children whose home environment has fostered tendencies towards moodiness, marked depression, and unhappiness through

[1] Grant, Samuel B., *Oxford Medicine*, VI, Part 2, 1927 Ed., p. 1101.

parental nagging or over-emotionality. Parental exaggeration of slight misbehaviour on the part of the child, severe punishment or threats of isolation which unduly terrify the child through imagination and horror of the unknown, have in some cases been known to produce a sudden onset of stuttering which has persisted long after the removal of the exciting cause.

Stuttering also seems to accompany the presence of enlarged glands such as hypertrophied tonsils and adenoids, probably due to the infiltration of toxic substances which affect the nerve centres in the brain and spinal cord. Anomalies of mouth, nose and throat seem to be factors which favour the development of habits of stuttering, as it is found in cases of high-arched palate, malformed epiglottis and short frenum. In these cases it is probably the sensitivity of the patient to this anomaly which leads to undue self-consciousness and to stuttering, rather than the anatomical peculiarity which is responsible for the onset of speech disturbances.

In severe stuttering there may be involvement of the muscles of lips, tongue, cheek, neck and shoulder muscles, and it may involve the limbs, particularly at the beginning of words, sentences or phrases.[1]

Kerley found that 35 per cent. of the stutterers whom he treated had had relatives who stuttered. Rogers found that the onset of stuttering often followed severe fright, traumatic shock, or childhood diseases.[2]

Stuttering is found among children who appear quite normal in all other respects ; it is also found among subnormal and deficient children ; it is found in superior children. The very diversity of the types among whom we find this disorder adds to our difficulty in ascertaining the exact causes. Not only is it found amid a wide variety of backgrounds, representing an extensive and complex etiology, but it yields to a great many varieties

[1] Kerley, *op. cit.*, p. 576.
[2] Rogers, J. F., *The Speech Defective School Child*, U.S. Dept. of the Interior, Bull. 7, 1931, 29 p.
*Ibid.*, *Speech Defects and Their Correction*, Pamphlet 22, 1931.

of treatment, ranging from that which emphasizes the physiological processes ; that which involves psychological methods primarily ; that which is chiefly suggestion with some " mental hygiene "—often not that which is advocated by psychiatrists themselves or recognized by them as such ; educational methods ; elocutionary drill ; speech correction with other groups of children in clinics ; private treatment in some commercially organized school for stammerers where usually there is little attention given to the medical and psychological principles involved, —and so on. There seems to be a greater diversity of treatment in this country than in Europe, as on the Continent and in England speech correction is still largely under medical control or supervision, whereas in this country it has been exploited by a wide variety of " specialists ", from the independent worker, the director of the special school for stammerers, to the educator, elocution teacher and the like. Only recently have any considerable number of physicians, dentists, psychologists, psychiatrists and educators become intensely interested in the field.

In studies compiled for the White House Conference in 1930, by West, Travis and Camp, they found that the median I.Q. for stutterers was 96·5 in a group of 4059 stutterers. This was higher than the I.Q. found for children having structural-articulatory defects, also for those having organic speech defects, and those having oral inaccuracies. The I.Q. found for those with sound substitutions was higher, as might be expected, than any of the others, or 98·2 I.Q. in a study of 6967 cases.[1]

The White House Conference Report found (1) that stuttering did not seem to be closely related etiologically to other disorders of speech ; (2) the survey found that stutterers were not mentally retarded ; (3) that more males stutter than females ; the ratio being 4 to 1 in a study of 10,268 cases ; (4) in the majority of cases, stuttering began before the age of six years.

[1] "The Handicapped Child ", White House Conference Proceedings, 1st Report, 1930, pp. 320–21.

There is a difference between a neurological and a neurotic disturbance in speech. In the case of aphasia we have a *real* impossibility, with an organic or a psychic disturbance, which prevents the speech mechanism from functioning. In stuttering we have an inhibition of a *possibility*, or a neurotic *inhibition of language*. There is a distinction between the non-possession of language and an inhibition of that which one possesses. In aphasia or dysphasia there is a reduction of psychical function ; in stuttering there may be no psychic loss, but merely a disturbance of utterance. According to the Freudian theory of language, the disturbance in speech is due to psychic conflicts and the inability to solve them ; the neurotic conflict finds expression in the speech disturbance. The material on which a patient stutters is therefore considered of special importance to the psycho-analyst, and is a possible field of research of considerable importance, as has been indicated by Freud in *The Psychopathology of Everyday Life*.

Delayed reaction-time and inhibition of speech gives to the psycho-analyst the immediate impression that there is resistance in the patient's mind, and that the inhibition is a form of protection against self-revelation in speech. This is an important " indicator ", therefore, according to the analyst.

The neurotic person is one who cannot tolerate with equanimity a displeasing situation. Intolerance versus displeasure in life situations is one indication of neurotic tendencies. Any conflict should lead to decision, but the neurotic cannot make decisions. He builds up a neurotic compromise, and the repressed material or repressed conflict, carried over into the unconscious or even into the subconscious mind, leads to " slips of speech ", to hesitation or to actual blocking at the attempt to initiate speech. Later, the speech hesitation having become an habitual reaction, the patient reacts by stuttering in any difficult situation in which speech is involved, particularly when it relates to himself, his own affairs or anything having an emotional significance for himself. In this he differs from the aphasic, according to recent theories, in that the aphasic *retains* words related to himself, his own activities, words having a signifying or an emotional function, but he loses or is inhibited in the utterance of words having an intellectual or an abstract import.

Karl Bühler has emphasized this fact in his discussion of the three functions of language, viz. :—

1. *Effeckvoll,* or *effective* language, given in order to secure a response from another individual.
2. *Expressive, subjective language,* characteristic of expression without reflection ; concrete language.
3. *Signifying* function of language, that which is intellectual or abstract.

In the background of every neurosis of childhood we find an infantile neurotic state to which it may be traced, according to the psycho-analyst. Neurotic anxiety often takes the form of a neurosis. The essential explanation of many a case of stuttering is therefore claimed by the analyst to be the persistence into adult life of infantile attitudes and conflicts for which the individual has not found a satisfactory solution. The principle of pleasure, struggling against the principle of reality, brings the mature individual into conflict, and this struggle may precipitate hesitation and speech blocking, according to this theory. One function of speech rehabilitation and of education is to replace the infantile attitude with an adult personality, in order to enable the individual to face reality squarely and courageously, and to attempt to find the solution for his particular problem. A president of the United States has said that there is no human problem which cannot be solved, if you can bring together the interested parties and persuade them to honestly and objectively face the situation, with a fair degree of give-and-take, and with a real desire to solve the problem in a fair way. This applies to personal and emotional, as well as to international conflicts.[1]

In the government hospital at Waukesha, Wisconsin,

[1] Hoover, Herbert E., *Radio Addresses.*

Blanton [1] found that among 100 war veterans with disorders of speech, hysteria led the list as the assigned cause for stuttering; anxiety-neuroses stood second; neurasthenia stood third; constitutional-psychopathic inferiority fourth; mental deficiency last.

Of 200 stuttering school children, aged five to eighteen years, studied by Blanton,[2] 13 per cent. showed no particular deviation from normal in their reactions; 52 per cent. showed marked feelings of inferiority; 35 per cent. were problem children because they were moody, unsocial, sulky, depressed or very excitable; 11 per cent. stuttered worse at school than at home.

In Wallin's survey of St. Louis school children, including some 98,000 subjects, he found 197 severe stutterers, 486 mild stutterers, 683 whose speech varied from mild to severe stuttering. The ratio was 3 boys to 1 girl among stutterers, but this ratio was not found for defects of speech other than stuttering.[3] Kenyon holds that the action of the oro-laryngeal muscles as a whole is quite dependent upon the mental *purpose* to produce a sound, and that such a sound, to be effective, must be restrained, directed by practice, and under the guidance of psychological control. Stuttering, he explains, occurs when there is too great a physiological tension in the peripheral speech musculature, or when the psychological control is crude, inadequate and poorly co-ordinated. This theory does not explain the *cause* of the hyper-tension, however.[4]

Twitmeyer [5] in his hemato-respiratory studies of stuttering, in the Psychological Laboratory of University of Pennsylvania, found that the breath-volume of stutterers was not below that of ordinary speakers, but was often higher. Robbins, in his studies of vaso-motor

[1] Blanton, S., " Speech Disorders as a Psychiatric Problem ", *Jour. A.M.A.*, 1921, 77, p. 375.

[2] Blanton, *op. cit.*

[3] Wallin, J. E., *Speech Defective Children in a Large School System.*

[4] Kenyon, E. L., " Action and Control of the Peripheral Organs of Speech ", *J.A.M.A.*, Nov. 3, 1929, pp. 1341–6.

[5] Twitmeyer, E. L., Univ. of Penna. Studies, " Hemato-respiratory Studies of Stutterers ", 1928–29.

variations in stutterers, using the pneumograph and plethysmograph, found increased vaso-motor activity in stutterers as compared with normal speakers.[1]

The first published biography of a stutterer is that of Wendall Johnson, University of Iowa, who describes the influence which a speech handicap has had upon his career, his interests and ambitions. He says: " An awkward tongue has moulded my life—and I have only one life to live. I shall try to tell you what it means to stutter—to describe the influences that it has had upon my personality, my ambitions, and my fundamental attitudes towards life." He writes in support of the cerebral-dominance theory.[2]

Studies of the action currents in stuttering have been reported by Orton and Travis [3] from the University of Iowa Laboratories. These studies having been devised to enable them to try to determine the native handedness of the individuals tested, by testing both sides of the body simultaneously. A control group of " normal " speakers, a group of ambidextrous subjects and a group consisting entirely of stutterers were used. They found that the action currents from the muscles of the right forearm preceded those from the left arm in most of the normal (right-handed) speakers. In the group of seventeen stutterers tested only three showed a greater number of right leads than left, and in two of these there were many " simultaneous leads ", or more than were found in the right-handed subjects.

Travis and Fagan made studies of certain reflexes during stuttering. Observation of the patellar and achilles reflexes during periods of silence and of speech were made.[4] They found that when the stutterer was speaking freely, there was, in contrast to the period of free speech

[1] Robbins, S. D., " A Plethysmographic Study of Shock and Stammering ", *Amer. Jour. of Physiology*, 48, 3, April 1919.

[2] Johnson, Wendall, *Because I Stutter*.

[3] " Studies in Stuttering ; IV, Action Currents in Stutterers ", *Arch. of Neurol. and Psychiatry*, Jan. 1929, 21, pp. 61–8.

[4] Travis-Fagan, " Studies in Stuttering ; Reflexes during Stuttering ", *Arch. of Neurol. and Psychiatry*, June 1928, 19, pp. 1006–13.

in right-handed subjects, a lesser amplitude recorded than during silent periods.

Kopp's studies of the bio-chemistry of stuttering, at University of Wisconsin,[1] promise to throw important light upon the physiological basis of this disorder. Influence of changes in blood chemistry, glands of internal secretion, food, diet, and other factors are compared in groups of subjects consisting of normal speakers and of stutterers.

Bluemel summarizes a large number of possible causes of stuttering, together with a wide variety of manifestations of the disorders such as respiratory symptoms, disturbances in vocalization, disturbances in articulation, facial contortions, combined symptoms, and varying degrees of severity. He finds the basis to be mental rather than physiological. He emphasizes the importance of unfavourable mental attitudes, undue excitement, unfortunate home conditions, and development of a personality which is conducive to feelings of inadequacy, insecurity, lack of self-confidence and over-dependence, in producing a setting which fosters the development of a speech defect such as we find in spasmophemia.

He finds that stammerers show muscular reactions in such activities as playing the piano or other musical instrument similar to those of the vocal organs in talking ; they also tend to stammer in writing and in other motor activities calling for manual dexterity. Stammering also occurs in typing and in telegraphing, in his subjects.

His method of treatment is described in detail and is one of the most lucid which we find in literature on the subject. The work for his subjects is roughly graded in classes according to age. Silent speech during which the child is required to make a mental preparation for overt speech is employed ; situations of an informal nature are created to favour ease of self-expression ; breathing is only touched upon incidentally, lest it foster muscle-consciousness and interfere with freedom of co-ordination

[1] Kopp, *Biochemical Studies of the Cause of Stuttering*, *pp.* 1–6, Symposium, 1932, Amer. Soc. for the Study of Dis. of Speech.

in a reflex activity. Relaxation exercises are given and are stressed with stutterers as a secondary aid to the establishment of ease in speaking, but as less important than clear thinking and the evolution of ideas to be expressed ; slow speech is not considered of particular importance, as the majority of normal speakers use a fairly rapid tempo, and it is to be recognized that the stutterer wishes to talk as normally as possible and in accordance with the customary manner of speaking which he hears about him. Individual conferences are given to the older pupils, as they are often able to make direct and immediate application of the suggestions given to aid their own progress. Encouragement and approbation are recognized by the instructor as fundamental to the progress of the patient. Assistance through group stimulation, talking with companions of one's own age, and the co-operation of parents are essential or advisable. Visual imagery is stressed as especially important in clearing up the mental confusion, chaotic condition accompanying efforts to speak, and as enabling the speaker to control his motor co-ordinations in speaking, through a careful patterning of his ideas in visual imagery. We may summarize Bluemel's contribution as the " transient visual amnesia " theory.[1]

Swift takes a somewhat similar view regarding the importance of imagery, but he stresses the transient auditory amnesia theory particularly, believing that the building up of adequate auditory images will remove chaotic speech impulses, lead to clear thinking, and to the control of the speech muscular processes in speaking.[2]

Fletcher gives an interesting plan for educational prophylaxis,[3] maintaining that the school should be the chief prophylactic agency, and that stuttering as a psychoneurosis must be considered as a problem for the school to solve through co-operation with medical and psychiatric agencies, within the school system. Horn [4] believes that

[1] Bluemel, C. S., *Mental Aspects of Stammering*, p. 152.
[2] Swift, W. B., *Speech Defects in School Children*.
[3] Fletcher, J., *The Problem of Stuttering*, 1928, pp. 320–23.
[4] Horn, J. L., *The Education of Exceptional Children*, 1929, Ch. IX.

I

special rooms or even special schools for stutterers and other speech-handicapped children should be established by public school authorities and universities. His plan if carried out, would call for part-time physicians, school nurses, psychiatric social-service workers, dental clinics, medical clinics, psychiatrists, full-time speech workers and part-time assistants who are interested in the speech-handicapped child to the same extent as they are now interested in the child with defects of vision or audition, or childhood diseases. Student assistants, trained in local universities, and co-operating with the teachers of speech correction, might well be considered in such a speech-education programme as Horn recommends, and it would take care of the financing of such a project, which seems at present to be the real obstacle to the inclusion of speech correction work in many school systems.

Russell, in his motion-picture studies of the vocal cords in action, has made it possible for us to demonstrate to any observer the activity which is taking place in the larynx during speech, and the way in which the vocal cords function normally, as compared with their inco-ordination and spasmodic action in stuttering and in certain diseased conditions.[1] Russell's invention of a laryngoscopic mirror by means of which one may demonstrate the vocal cords in action, has made it possible for the teacher and student to actually see what is taking place in any larynx during speech activity.

Brown [2] holds that stuttering is a neurophysiological disorder, and that the seat of the disturbance is possibly the optic thalamus, where a delay may occur in the process of transmission of speech impulses, as the thalamus is now believed to be the seat of emotional impulses. The occurrence of ideas surcharged with emotion, or in which there are conflicting impulses making clear decisions difficult, and in which there is undue strain, anxiety or

[1] Russell, J. O., *Ohio State University Researches*, " Motion Picture Studies ". *Ibid.*, *The Vowel*.

[2] Brown, F., " Viewpoints on Stuttering ", *Am. J. Orthopsychiatry*, 2, Jan. 1932.

nervous tension, tends to obstruct the transmission of impulses from the word-memory centres to the motor-speech mechanism, through obstruction within the thalamus. The inhibitory influence, according to Brown,[1] takes place within the sensory speech areas, and prevents the transmission of the necessary impulses over the association fibres, to the motor centres of the brain. A motor " stop-signal " is thus given to the motor mechanism, by the sensory areas of the brain. This implies a subcortical or associative inhibition of speech, and agrees more or less with the earlier findings of neurologists regarding the associative aphasias. Fröschels, following the European investigators on aphasia, speaks of stuttering as a form of *associative aphasia*, and believes that it is only another manifestation of some type of functional aphasia.[1] This is also the viewpoint of Hoepfner, another European investigator. Fröschels finds four stages in stuttering, in any one of which the patient may be at the time of examination, depending upon how long or with what severity he has stuttered.[2] There is the *clonic* stage with a mere repetition of syllables, as " d–d–d–do you want ? "—etc. Measurements of time or repetition show that such syllables take no more time than ordinary speech, and the fact that it has the *same tempo* is against the theory that it can be a *true cramp*. The second stage is a *klono-tonus* [3] state, in which the patient begins to employ laboured or forced expulsion of tone ; strong blocking occurs, especially forceful utterance being used on the opening sound or word, as *P*-apa, for pa*pá*. In this stage the child may become a real stutterer. He feels that words are difficult, and that to do that which is difficult, one must exert force, and so he labours desperately to produce the desired effect in speech, and in the effort the speech becomes slower than usual.

The third stage is called by Fröschels that of *embolo-*

[1] Brown, F., "Viewpoints on Stuttering", *Am. J. Orthopsychiatry*, 2, Jan. 1932.

[2] Fröschels, E., *Das Stottern (assoziativ Aphasie)*, 1925.

[3] Klonus—the vibratory, or repetitious movement, as in repetition of sounds like p–p–p–, or m–m–m– before finishing the word.

*phrasia*, in which the concomitant movements appear, along with speech blocking. Facial muscles, arms, legs, head and neck muscles may become abnormally strained, tense or chaotic during the effort to speak. The child may then employ helping sounds, speech noises or mannerisms and meaningless sounds. There may be a *tono-clonus* at this time [1] and a tendency to speak faster than in stage two.

The final stage is that of *concealment*, in which the patient tries to hide his difficulty either through employing concomitant movements which are scarcely perceptible, such as slight facial tics or habit-spasms which enable him to start his speech, but which do not always reveal him immediately as a stutterer. It is easier to cure the stutterer of his difficulty in the earlier than in the later stages, according to Fröschels, who stresses the importance of corrective measures in childhood.

Fröschels' treatment is based upon the assumption that one can treat "states of illness" in speech with knowledge and understanding, just as one might expect to treat patients presenting definite pathological symptoms, but that the therapy should be very different. The patient must be shown that the situations which he fears are actually not difficult to meet, that his own personal problems are capable of solution, and that there is no foundation in fact for his dread of speech situations. The stutterer must first be treated by psychological methods, in other words, his attitude towards environment, and towards himself and society, must be changed. He must feel that he needs to do things quietly and smoothly, even though some things are more difficult and necessarily require more effort than others ; he must be taught that there is a normal solution for every problem ; that he must seek the normal way to express himself quietly, without effort or without concomitant muscle

---

[1] Tonus—the contraction of muscles of speech, adding force or great effort to the speech impulse. (Cf. with tonic-spasm.)

Tono-clonus, and clono-tonus, a combination of the two, the order in which they seem to take place, determining the term used.

movements and facial contortions, as this is not normal. One must get at the psychic foundation for the speech defect, as well as to try to remedy the accidental speech symptoms.

*Treatment Summarized.*—Whatever is conducive to stabilizing the nervous system of the child or adult, whether the means be psychotherapy, physiotherapy or a combination of both, is important in the treatment of this speech disorder. Suggestion plays an important part, particularly in hysterical or suggestible individuals and in children. In strong-willed, aggressive or negatively-suggestible children such methods must be more subtly used, to secure results favourable to the patient. Measures to re-establish self-confidence must be included. Emphasis should be upon the purpose of speech, the ideas and intention of the speaker, rather than primarily upon elocutionary " drills " outward manifestations, phonetics or the repetition of speech sounds. Calling the attention to any reflex activity interferes with the smoothness of response. Calling attention to the disorder called stuttering, in its incipient stages, may tend to fixate the habit rather than to facilitate its removal. After such a habit has become set, the calling of attention to the act and forcing the stutterer to reproduce his facial grimaces and concomitant muscle movements voluntarily, has been found to be very successful as a method of curing such unfavourable acquired speech tendencies, according to Dunlap. Since stuttering " spasms " are not true spasms, they cannot be true reflexes, but rather habit spasms, or muscle movements accompanying the speech impulse, which may be brought under voluntary control, if one is successful in finding the appropriate method to fit the individual case.[1]

The European speech clinics have been more cautious in the application of psycho-analysis to the cure of stuttering, than have American and English workers, but in the clinics after the Freudian, Jung and Adlerian schools, many cures are reported following the use of the

[1] Dunlap, *op. cit.*

psycho-analytic method.  Those forms of psycho-analysis which take into account both the psychic and the physical states, and which are sufficiently broad as to include other than sex-complexes as the primary causative factor, and which supply the speech worker with an adequate knowledge of the case in hand through well-systematized and complete case histories, physical and neurological findings, psychiatric study and psychological tests, seem most fruitful of results, according to the author's experience and belief.

DYSPHONIA

Dysphonia may be defined as any defect of voice due to morbid condition of the larynx or its immediate innervation, to defective respiration, to anomalies in the resonance cavities of the throat, mouth or nose, or to dysfunction causing an alteration in the vocal quality, or an inability to phonate.

In cases of temporary loss of voice there is frequently an acute inflammatory condition of the larynx.  In temporary loss of voice the physician often finds that enlarged tonsils or adenoids, or both, have caused the inflammatory condition by infiltration or discharge of toxic substances from the oral or nasal cavity into the throat.  When only the false cords are affected, a condition known as " croup " results, with vocal hoarseness.  When the inflammatory condition includes the vocal cords themselves, laryngitis usually results, with temporary loss of voice.  In cases where one or both of the vocal cords have been removed, or a cancerous condition has been treated, the voice has a " croup-like " characteristic, which sounds like a hypophonia or forcing of tone.

Laryngitis does not always disappear permanently, with the removal of tonsils and adenoids.  Singers and public speakers, after the removal of diseased tissue, often find that if they are forced to use the voice under conditions of undue strain and fatigue, hypophonia may result.

Mary R., following a severe attack of whooping-cough,

was unable to phonate above a hoarse whisper. After some practice she was able to make herself heard through the class-room, in a whispered voice. As seen through the laryngoscope, her vocal cords appeared to be swollen and permanently enlarged, with edges thickened, so that normal approximation and vibration for voiced sounds was impossible.

Absence of speech is rarely due to malformations of the organs of speech. It may be due to a temporary organic condition which renders vocalization impossible, or may appear following or accompanying various diseases, the voice returning to its normal condition when the diseased condition has cleared up.

The usual procedure, with children, is to attend to the removal of diseased tonsils or adenoids when the condition is such as to threaten the child's health, and when he is subject to frequent respiratory diseases. Hay fever brings with it an inflammatory condition of the nostrils which affects the voice much like a heavy " cold ". Immunization of children for this common disorder often brings seasonal relief. Adult singers and speakers need to exercise good mouth and throat hygiene, especially when they are prone to respiratory infections. If parents were insistent upon the exercise of proper care of mouth, throat and nose in childhood, many adults would be free from the annoyances caused by respiratory infections in later life. We still fail to realize that a succession of light or heavy " colds " in winter is unhygienic and to some extent preventable.

### Common Laryngeal Diseases associated with Hoarseness and Loss of Voice

#### Croup

This is characterized by a dry, harsh " barking " cough. It is usually associated with respiratory obstruction, hypertrophied tonsils or adenoid tissue. Laryngeal spasms and difficult breathing occur with increased pulse beat. In severe cases there is a loud, crowing sound in inspiration.   The hoarseness may persist into the daytime, but is usually worst at night.

## Traumatic Laryngitis

This is often produced by the inhalation of strong gases or steam, or by the aspiring of strong acids.   During the World War, the inhalation of poisonous gases caused a loss of voice which was usually temporary, but which was, in some cases, permanent.

## Laryngeal Obstruction

Following croup this condition often appears.   It may be due to laryngismus stridulus, to inflammation of the larynx, traumatic laryngitis, or to abscesses posterior to the pharynx.   It may cause partial or complete obstruction to respiration.

## Laryngismus Stridulus

In this disease spasms of the larynx involve the muscles of inspiration and of expiration.   It usually occurs before the eighteenth month of infancy, and is frequently found in rachitic children or others who are poorly nourished. It may be induced by violent emotional states.   The thymus is sometimes involved.   Although no definite lesion has been found, in this disease, it occurs with many morbid states.   It is characterized by a sudden onset of difficult breathing which alternates with periods of normal respiration.   The prognosis is good with improved nutrition and in case the thymus gland is not involved.   Good physical care, freedom from over-exertion and excitement, freedom from nagging or rough treatment by other children or adults should be insisted upon during the course of this disease, and in all children who are prone to such attacks.[1]

## Postadenoidal Speech

Hypertrophy of adenoid tissue causes a compensatory widening of the posterior nares, according to Glassburg,

[1] Kerley, *op. cit.*, pp. 537–39.

and when this is curetted, there may be too much space for a complete closure of soft palate, uvula and tongue during phonation. The result is a peculiar nasal tone. Sometimes this condition is corrected easily by vocal training, but if the space is too wide, training is ineffective, and all except the nasal sounds are over-nasalized. The speech sounds muffled, and in order to secure greater clearness it is necessary to re-educate the muscles controlling the soft palate, velum and back of the tongue.

The following is a summary of some of the exercises given in such cases.

## EXERCISES

1. Ask the patient to throw the head back, and to say " ah–h–h–rah " several times. Observe whether the velum occludes the posterior nares.

2. Have patient extend tongue forward and downwards toward chin.

3. Extend tongue outward and upward as far as possible.

4. Point tongue alternately upwards and downwards for 10 counts.

5. Rotate tongue to right and down ; then to left and upwards.

6. Protrude tongue, groving it by raising sides.

7. With mouth open, curl tip of tongue back of front teeth.

8. Press tip of tongue to back of the front teeth ; then relax.

## LIP EXERCISES

1. Pucker the lips and protrude them.

2. Raise the upper lip, exposing upper teeth.

3. Wrinkle the nose so as to expose the upper teeth.

4. Raise right side of upper lip.

5. Raise left side of upper lip.

6. Pull lower lip down, exposing lower teeth.

## SOFT PALATE AND UVULA EXERCISES

1. With mouth open, say " ah–ng–ah–ng–ah–ng–ah " several times. Observe action of tongue and velum.

2. Yawn and watch palate rise.

3. Practise " ah " sounds several times, and alternate with nasal sounds such as " ah–ung–ah ;   ee–hung–ee ; oh–ung–oh ;  oo–ung–oo ", etc.

### *Paraphonia or Morbid Alterations of Voice—Glands of Internal Secretion*

In many diseases we find speech defects which are closely associated with the deficiency or with the hyper-activity of glands of internal secretion.   This may be easily demonstrated in characteristic vocal signs or symptoms which we find in various cases of mental deficiency, in psychoses and in some of the psychoneuroses.   Thyroid deficiency, for instance, not only is responsible for stunted mental and physical development, but the mental torpor is apparent in the speech reactions of the individual, and in the quality of vocal responses, as compared with normal speech.[1]

Hyper-secretion of the thyroid glands causes an effect quite contrary to that produced by a deficiency.   Mental activity is often unduly stimulated, over-emotionality and behaviour disorders may appear, the speech-pressure may become such that the tempo is rapid, cluttered and hasty. The excessive nervous energy consumed tends toward a wasting of strength, lack of poise and unbalance.   This is frequently apparent in the voice and personality of the speaker.

L. was an exopthalmic-goitre case, with occasional stuttering.   While the speech defect was mild, the weakness in character was apparent in many of the avoidance reactions made by the student.   He always avoided meeting difficulties squarely, and in the attempt to escape responsibility became involved in a serious disciplinary affair in his university, which threatened to cut short his college career.   The only physiological basis for the stuttering seemed to be hyper-thyroidism.   How much of

[1] Blanton, *Speech Training for Children*, Century Co., N.Y., 1919. *Ibid., Child Guidance*, N.Y., 1928.

this was responsible for his hyper-emotionality, character defect and flabbiness of will, is largely a matter of speculation. That there was a relationship was probable.

## Spasmophilia and Latent Tetany

Spasmophilia is the name applied to that form of disease known as latent tetany. It is characterized by nervous irritability in infants. Such symptoms as holding the breath, convulsions, carpo-pedal spasms and laryngospasms are common. It appears most frequently in bottle-fed infants after about the third month. Deficiency of lime salts or toxic condition of the system following contagious disease or digestive disturbance are causative factors. The laryngospasm is present in crying or upon slight nervous excitation. Treatment is much the same as in rickets. The significance of its connection with speech disorders is, that it appears in stuttering and that Chvostek's sign often is present and may remain as an habitual pattern reaction during speech even after the patient ceases to stutter.

Suggestion and psychotherapy play an important part in curing such disorders and in restoring the voice to its normal condition. Home treatment of a quiet, orderly, non-nagging type is desirable. Severe punishment should be avoided. Even severe threats by parents or nurses may increase the nervous tension, quicken the speech tempo, and cause characteristic signs of nervousness to become a part of the usual speech reaction. Hysterical symptoms usually yield to the right sort of treatment, including the avoidance of over-dramatizing the situation or condition, and not allowing the child to " play to a gallery." Parents should use good sense, adopt a casual attitude, distract the child's attention by some unusual stimulus or incident, until they succeed in modifying the first reaction into a more desirable one. Rest, sleep, supervision of play-time, and a restful environment are the best sedatives for nervous children.[1]

[1] Kerley, *Practice of Pediatrics*, pp. 540–547.

Experiments at University of Wisconsin [1] indicate that tetany, infantile convulsions and spasmophilia can be produced and stopped at will. Certain toxins, or a calcium deficiency or disturbed acid-base, can be made to produce tetany experimentally.[2] C. R. Stockard and others have demonstrated that castration causes vocal changes. Later experiments have shown that the voice is restored to its normal pitch if certain hormones are injected into the blood stream, following post-pubertal castration. G. H. Parker [3] maintains that the nerves of the body secrete a substance at the terminal end, or end-brush. He believes that this secretion at the synopses of the nervous system may cause delay in transmission of a nerve impulse, as in speech disturbances.

*Rickets.*—Rachitic children are known to have inhibitory control of a lower order than non-rachitic children. The nerve centres seem to share with other portions of the body the malnutrition and atypical development. Mild irritation is enough to induce convulsive seizures or similar reactions in rachitic children. This is a possible factor in the etiology of facial grimaces, tics, habit spasms and stuttering, as well as in oral inaccuracy and generally ineffective speech.

The lack of Vitamines A and D in the diet has been found to be the cause of rickets, and if children are fed rations lacking in these vitamines, and if they are deprived of fresh air and sunshine, they tend to become rachitic. Disparity between the size of the head and of the rest of the body or of the extremities in children who have had rickets, is an important indicator. Rickets also affects dental development rather often, due to the deficiency in salts. Jaw malformation and poorly developed teeth often result.[4]

[1] Kopp, *Bio-Chemical Studies of the Cause of Stuttering*, Amer. Soc. for the Study of Disorders of Speech, Papers, 1931, pp. 1–6.

[2] MacLeod, *Physiology and Bio-Chemistry in Modern Medicine*, p. 1016.

[3] Parker, *The Collecting Net*, Publica. Researches, Woods Hole, N.Y.

[4] Smiley and Gould, *College Textbook of Hygiene*, 1928.

# CHAPTER VII

## DYSLOGIA AND DYSPHASIA

### TYPICAL CASE STUDIES

#### DYSLOGIA

DYSLOGIA is defined as difficulty in vocal expression of ideas in speech, due to impairment of reasoning power in psychoses and feeble-mindedness.  The Dyslogias constitute an important part of work in speech correction, and it is often very difficult to differentiate between a mildly neurotic or poorly adjusted personality, and one in which mental deterioration has reached an advanced stage.  Because such cases are often referred to the speech pathologist or speech clinical worker, it is worth while to spend some time in reviewing the more important types of nervous disorders, in order to better understand their implications, in undertaking speech therapy.

Dyslogia occurs in connection with various types of psychoses and in certain psychoneuroses.  The main forms are summarized as follows :—

1. Agrammalogia or incoherent speech.
2. Alogia, or absence of ideas.
3. Anarthrialogia ; loss of power of expression ; slurring speech.[1]
4. Aphasialogia ; mental impairment due to lesion or to disturbances in association and integration.[1]
5. Bradylogia or sluggish speech.
6. Catalogia—verbigeration.
7. Paralogia—irrelevant speech.
8. Polylogia—logorrhea.

[1] Given in unpublished revision, Robbins-Stinchfield *Dictionary*, *op. cit.*, p. 5.

## The Psychoneuroses and Speech Disturbances

Speech disorders are frequently one of the first diagnostic signs apparent to the psychiatrist in various types of mental disorder.   While the speech deterioration or impairment may be mild or severe, according to the nature of the mental disorder, suddenness and severity of the attack and other factors, it is often an aid to the physician and to the speech pathologist, to whom such cases are sometimes referred before they are recognized as indicative of a psychoneurosis or of a psychosis.

## The Psychoneuroses

Anarthrialogia or loss of power of expression, disturbances in articulation, slurring of syllables or words, and various forms of aphasia or aphasialogia are among the chief types of speech defect in hysteria, neurasthenia and psychasthenia.   They are also found in anxiety states or anxiety neuroses, but the above-named types are the chief forms of psychoneuroses.   Incoherent speech, absence of ideas, repetitious speech, irrelevant speech and logorrhea or speech pressure are found in various milder hysterical states, but are more apparent in the psychoses, such as in manic depressive insanity, and dementia præcox.

## Hysteria

Hysteria is a form of psychoneurosis manifesting itself in countless disturbances of the psychic, sensory, motor or vasomotor functions.   It is sometimes described as the " conversion of a mental shock into a physical symptom ".   According to Rosanoff [1] it is not a disease but a temperamental abnormality for which there is no organic basis.   The range of symptoms manifested is extensive and may simulate any one of a number of different diseases.   The symptoms are such as may be produced at will.

Hysterical mutism is frequently mentioned in the literature which has appeared since the World War, in

[1] Rosanoff, A., *Manual of Psychiatry*, 1927.

the writings of such authors as Pierre Janet, Southard, Rosanoff, Blanton and others. Sudden shock occurs, and the patient finds himself temporarily unable to speak. He may lose power of speech for several hours or for days, due to the persistence of the traumatic state. Recovery usually follows rest, electro-therapy, suggestion and medical treatment.

Freud traces all hysterias to a neuropathic background, and believes that the condition has its origin in the sex life of the individual. Jung has made important analyses of the speech content of individuals suffering from various psychoneuroses, and supports Freud's views in part, but he finds other bases for abnormal behaviour in the cases studied. According to Rosanoff,[1] hysteria is a character defect, and its manifestation is the result of a concealed ethically inferior motive.

During hysterical seizures of the spasmodic variety, the lips and tongue are often involved and facial spasms appear. Absence of speech or aphonia may cover a long period of time, or may occur for short intervals, or intermittently, alternating with periods in which the speech is normal. According to Southard the occurrence of hysterical mutism among soldiers during the World War was very frequent. In most of the cases a neuropathic background or neuropathic taint appeared in the case history. When speech returned it was often in the form of a severe stutter, which gradually improved under rest, therapy and hospitalization.

Golla found that in the hysteric the bodily changes accompanying emotion were abnormal. Using the psychogalvanic test of Veraguth, he found that the emotive reaction was markedly depressed in his subjects.[2] Further experiments with the plethysmograph and the pneumograph showed the emotional reactions of the hysteric to be subnormal. He found that the patient tended to dramatize some internal conflict through pseudo-pathological forms of expression.

[1] Rosanoff, A., *op. cit.*
[2] Golla, *Oxford Medicine*, VI, Part 2, pp. 999–1025.

The symptoms which the hysteric chooses for expression assume increasing importance for him, and may be easily reinforced by overmuch sympathy or concern. Like the true actor, the hysteric must play to a gallery. French neurologists attribute the persistence of hysteria in patients to the desire to suppress painful memories, and to divert them from unpleasant experiences, rather than to the presence of repressed " complexes " of the Freudian type.

*Prognosis.*—Psychotherapy and suggestion are among the most effective measures in treatment. The psychology of suggestion must be very subtly given, else it may work havoc with the patient, however. A study of the " repressed complexes " is held by some neurologists to be less effective than a study of association responses made to some such objective test as the Jung word-association test. Delayed reaction time, quality of the response, variations in responses given on repetition and attitude of the patient during such a test are important indicators. One must try to uproot the unfortunate system of ideas which dominates the mind of the patient to an abnormal degree. This is sometimes done by shock or surprise methods, by unusual treatment, electro-therapy, or vigorous exercise, in all of which suggestion plays an important part. There is a danger of treating symptoms instead of causes in hysteria. Frequent treatment by the same person, whether by verbal suggestion, physiotherapy, psychotherapy, mental hygiene, or analysis often leads to the establishment of an atmosphere of cure, and to successful results.

### Psychasthenia

*Condition and Causes.*—This type of nervous disorder is characterized by abnormal impulses or fears and obsessions. It may take the form of abnormal fear of infections or of disease ; fear of objects ; fear of certain words ; or the patient may be tortured by doubts and indecision. Sometimes the symbolic words or objects cause so much pain to the patient, that in the attempt to remove them, the patient is pushed beyond endurance or even to suicide.

Janet describes this disorder as one in which one finds obsessions, phobias, states of hesitation, doubt and great anxiety. Compulsive ideas, subjective feelings of deficiency, psychological deficiencies and physiological disturbances are common. The patient finds insuperable obstacles in the affairs of everyday life. There is a decreased power of mind to adapt itself to ordinary requirements. Janet holds that there are two forms— hereditary and acquired. The first is the more serious, and may appear at any age, recovery being questionable. The second may appear at any age, but usually follows some disease, shock or strain. The latter is usually of short duration and cures are easily effected. Déjerine maintains that hysteria and neurasthenia are of psychogenic origin but that psychasthenia is not.[1]

Freud finds the psychoneurotic symptom to be a symbol of repressed psychic forces which have been forced back into the unconscious, because they are not acceptable to consciousness, and must therefore appear in disguised or in indirect form. The indirect outlet for the repressed force is found in psychasthenia.

*Speech.*—The chief characteristic of speech in this disturbance is not so much the presence of any particular " defect ", as a quality of speech, or speech content which reveals the mental state of the patient. Psychoanalysis was the method devised by Freud for investigation and treatment of the psychoneuroses. The technique is difficult and the treatment long and expensive. It should be used only by a trained psychoanalyst. Janet devised a simpler method, called the " director " method, by means of which the patient found that his activities were to be guided by the advice and suggestions of his physician, who should take upon himself the burdens of the patient and thus simplify reality for him.

[1] Hart, B., " Psychasthenia ", *Oxford Medicine*, VI, Part 2, pp. 1045–64.

K

## Neurasthenia

*Condition and Causes.*—Neurasthenia is the milder form of the psychoneuroses. It nearly approaches so-called normal behaviour. According to Moebius, it is the original source from which may be derived hysteria, hypochondria, melancholia and insanity. Although slight at the start, it sometimes is the forerunner of a serious disorder terminating in a psychosis. One finds in the neurasthenic a combination of various mental stigmata, chief of which are nervous exhaustion, tendency to tire easily, nerve weakness, poor endurance, hypochondriasis and constitutional flabbiness of musculature. Long-continued effort or exertion is not usual in these cases. The asthenia is not limited to muscular weakness. The patient is intellectually in the same condition as he is in regard to physical exertion. He cannot read for any length of time, cannot concentrate, and any slight effort may bring on headache, neuralgia or insomnia. The muscular flabbiness often leads to digestive disturbances, palpitation, and unusual sensory disturbances which render the patient gloomy and irritable. Asthenia also is found in the moral domain. The " insufficiency of potentiality " shows itself in the functioning of the entire being, the powerlessness being physical, intellectual and moral.[1]

*Prognosis and Treatment.*—The treatment is much the same as that for psychasthenia and hysteria. Psychiatric advice is usually given, and treatment is given to improve the muscle tonus and to secure the patient's co-operation in improving his general physical condition. Treatment of symptoms is not usually permanently effective, unless one also attempts to analyse the patient's psychic state and to try to remove sources of irritation, or to simplify the environment until the condition of the patient has improved. Speech teacher and psychiatrist may sometimes co-operate in the cure.

[1] Dubois, P., *Psychic Treatment of Nervous Disorders*, 1909.

*Morbid Fears ; Anxiety Neuroses* [1]

Functional mental disturbances in children are rare as compared with adults. When present they generally indicate an unfavourable heredity or very unfavourable environment. Abnormal fears and anxiety states are often assigned as causes of stuttering.

A young woman recently reported that the onset of stuttering in her case dated quite clearly to the day when her mother shut her in a large closet, as a punishment for some minor misbehaviour. She began to stutter violently, when released, and although the stuttering became intermittent, she was subject to stuttering at the time when she entered college. During a year of speech corrective training, during which she was brought to face her difficulty intelligently, she began to overcome her fear of speech situations. The nervous tension and fear present in the original situation, which had caused her difficulty, had come to be symbolic, and reappeared in any difficult situation or in any which involved social adjustments, conversation, and taking initiative.

Therapy was mainly through suggestion, analysis of the cause of her difficulty, facing the situation squarely, and then training the vocal mechanism through occasional practice in reading, participation in social situations, conversations, story-telling and improved socialization. The girl showed marked improvement by the end of her freshman year in college.

The hysterical stutterer improves more rapidly than do stutterers of a different temperament, usually, as has been noted by Blanton and others. Undoubtedly many of the so-called " cures " are recruited from the ranks of the hysterical stutterer who is somewhat suggestible and who therefore yields readily to treatment.

*The Psychoses*

It is not within the scope or intention of this volume to discuss the psychoses in detail. We shall confine

[1] Reference should also be made to Chap. VI., *Dysphemia*.

ourselves to the two most common types of dementia, to illustrate certain speech disturbances which occur in many of the psychoses, and which are often accompanied by rather important speech symptoms with which the speech pathologist should be familiar. Dementia Præcox and Manic Depressive Insanities, in their various forms, show marked deterioration in speech, as the mind becomes impaired. These speech symptoms are of diagnostic value to the physician and to the speech clinician.[1]

## Dementia Præcox

*Condition and Causes.*—Dementia Præcox is not usually found in early childhood, but around the twelfth year. It is often preceded by neurasthenia or by hysterical symptoms. The common types are (1) the hebephrenic, (2) the catatonic, and (3) the paranoic. Kraepelin assigns 14 to 15 per cent. of all admissions to asylums to this disease. It is equally common in men and women.

Among the causes cited are unfavourable heredity and auto-intoxication following various diseases of a severe infectious nature. There is some chemical injury to the cortical cells of the brain. Jung asserts that many cases are of a psychogenic origin and that the toxic condition may be induced as a result of rigidly repressed complexes, hyper-emotionality and distorted or warped systems of ideas leading to chemical damage and involving destruction of cortical cells.

While orientation may not be disturbed, illusions and hallucinations are present, especially of the auditory type. They sometimes arouse the patient to irritation or anger, or may merely amuse him by their supposed " import ". Memory is little affected. The common speech symptom is stereotyped language, irrelevance or incoherence in the expression of ideas, senseless repetitions, rhyming, punning and other forms of verbigeration.[2]

Emotional deterioration is present, indifference or apathy

---

[1] White, Wm., *Outlines of Psychiatry.*
[2] Franz, S. I., *Nervous and Mental Re-education.*

replace former interests and activities. Echolalia and mutism may alternate with one another. At other times the speech may appear quite normal. Stransky has been credited with the theory of " intrapsychic ataxia ", in which he attributed peculiarities in emotional expression and thinking to inco-ordination between mental and emotional life.

*Prognosis.*—The prognosis in dementia præcox is rather unfavourable. Recovery occurs, but the chances for complete recovery are less than in many other types of psychoses. The chances for recovery depend upon severity of the disorder, conditioning factors in the environment, heredity and type of response made by the patient to therapeutic measures. To deal merely with the speech disorder, in this disease, is to treat merely a symptom, and is of little value. The speech worker, if she suspects a serious underlying mental derangement when such a patient has been referred to her, should work from the standpoint of mental hygiene and mental therapy, and under the direction of the psychiatrist, merely as a means to the possible attainment of a normal psychic state by the patient.

## Manic Depressive Insanity

*Condition and Causes.*—Manic depressive insanity is often called circular insanity, because of the alternation of manic and depressive phases. According to Kraepelin about 8 per cent. of these cases show an hereditary basis. While it usually does not appear before the twenty-fifth year, it may occur as early as the tenth. The speech signs during the manic phase are undue verbiage, marked elation, flight of ideas, irrelevancy and general speech pressure. Hallucinations and illusions occur ; the ideas are connected, but often repeated, and rhyming, punning speech is common. There is loss of control of inhibitory ideas and this appears in the patient's use of unusual forms of expression, coprolalia and the like. There is great distractibility but no paralysis and no true anæsthesia.

The temperature is usually about normal. During the depressive phase there is retardation in thinking, motor inhibition and dejection. Hallucinations of a painful character are present and delusions are common. The patient may pay no attention to remarks addressed to him, and may reply in an inaudible whisper or may remain mute.

*Prognosis.*—About 70 per cent. of the patients recover from this disease. The prognosis is better than in the case of Dementia Præcox. Here, again, to treat merely the speech, is to treat only a symptom. If speech work is attempted, it should only be as a form of distraction to interest the patient and to re-orient him into normal mental interests, if this is possible. The speech teacher who suspects any such mental deviation on the part of a speech patient referred to her, should hasten to communicate with a psychiatrist, before the disorder has reached an advanced stage. An illustration of a typical case occurring in a college community serves to illustrate our point.

### Case A

A young college woman of twenty-four suddenly exhibited marked signs of unusual behaviour and speech. At first her companions were concerned solely with the peculiar content of her speech. During the opening week of college she showed marked tendencies to disagree with her instructors, argued violently but logically in class, and at the end of four days asked one of the professors to look over her " manuscript " about which her " publishers had telegraphed her several times ". Her pen-name was an assumed masculine cognomen. During the week she quarrelled violently with the clergyman who called to see her and she insulted the physician who was called in on the case. She kept her housemates in a turmoil for several days and nights before her condition was recognized as serious. Her speech during this time was normal in sound and quality of voice, but misrepresentations, delusions and hallucinations occurred and were obvious from her speech. Verbigeration, incoherent speech, flight of ideas occurred alternating with periods of lucidity. The illusion of being a prophet indicated the paranoid trend of her thinking. She reacted adversely to the presence of members of her family, and would respond only to two members of the faculty who were recent acquaintances.

That there was some insight into her condition was apparent from her remarks at various times. For two days it was possible to quiet her by appealing to her religious tendencies, as she had been educated in the Catholic Church, and the mere repetition of a Latin chant served to quiet her for moments at a time, during which she recited certain chants herself. This sufficed for only a short time, however, and eventually broke down entirely.

In this case it was the unusual substance of the speech reactions, unusual mental activities and verbosity, which attracted the attention of her housemates to her serious condition. The main basis for her response to the psychologist who stayed with her until a psychiatrist arrived, was a common bond of literary interest. Her speech in the beginning of her disturbance was indicative of a thwarted craving which was one basis for her serious mental state. She had desired intensely to do literary work, and was a great admirer of a relative who had associated herself with a publishing house. She herself had wished to undertake a similar occupation but had been thwarted by her family, who insisted that she enter the teaching profession. She found teaching in a mill-community very distasteful, discipline difficult, and the work not at all to her taste. Her breakdown followed a hectic, nerve-racking year of teaching under more than ordinarily difficult conditions. It is possible that a better understanding of her temperament and interests might have prevented a complete breakdown, at least until later life. The prognosis was poor, however, due to unfavourable heredity and mental instability in both the paternal and maternal ancestry, both in the direct and in collateral lines of descent.

## Dysphasia

Dysphasia is defined as a weakening or loss of power of forming language associations in any of its forms, such as in writing, speaking, or in comprehension of the written, printed or spoken word, due to impaired mental imagery, difficulty in re-forming associations previously acquired or in the combination of ideas and reactions in the various forms of expression. The forms of dysphasia which are due to organic lesions occur in many types of disease which have been discussed under Dysarthria, to which they are closely related. The forms of dysphasia which belong to the associative type are scarcely to be grouped with the dysarthrias. The student of speech should compare the various forms of dysphasia with the dysarthrias discussed in Chapter V, and with Dysphemia, as discussed in Chapter VI.

### Historical Theories as to the Conditions and Causes of Dysphasia

Dysphasia is usually referred to in the older literature as aphasia, which means literally *without speech*. The more recent term *dysphasia* is used in this chapter, as being more accurate. Since Broca's discovery in 1864, that " aphasia " resulted from injury to the third, left, frontal convolution of the brain, in right-handed persons, many studies of this disorder have been made, to determine the exact location of lesions responsible for sensory and motor disturbances of speech. The theory of localization seemed to be further confirmed by Wernicke's demonstration of the involvement of the left superior temporal gyrus in acoustic-sensory aphasia.

### Modern Conceptions regarding Aphasia

Recent theories tend to discard the grammatical and anatomical distinctions of a generation ago, in which three kinds of aphasia were postulated, namely, motor, sensory, mixed and total. In sensory aphasia it was believed that when the lesion was in the visual area, the understanding of words seen or read was lost, and that the patient became word-blind as a result. If the lesion was in the auditory centre, auditory word-memories were lost, and the patient became word-deaf. If the writing-centre was injured, in the motor area of the brain, the patient was unable to recall motor-writing patterns, or to write from dictation.[1] If the injury or lesion was in Broca's area, the patient was unable to recall the motor movements associated with speech, and speech was lost, or jargon speech was substituted. Destruction of both motor and sensory areas was held accountable for total aphasia.

Until recently, the most widely accepted theories of aphasia were those of Pierre Marie and of Head, the European investigators. Head postulated the following types of aphasic disturbances :—

1. Verbal aphasia in which recognition of word-meanings is lost or impaired. The patient cannot read or cannot understand printed words.

2. Nominal aphasia in which words and symbols have lost their meaning, reading and writing being impaired, and the ability to copy printed symbols being lost.

3. Syntactical aphasia, in which spoken words have lost their meaning. The patient tends towards jargon speech and incoherent utterance.

4. Semantic aphasia, in which comprehension of meanings is lost, as a whole, although separate words may be understood. Writing, reading, and comprehension of figures is little impaired.

According to Marie, there are no specific reading, writing and speech " centres ". He believes that the seat of the disturbance is in the supramarginal, angular and posterior region of the upper temporal gyri. This is known as Wernicke's Sensory Aphasia, which is cortical, and in which the intellect is impaired. When the lesion is in the lenticular zone, which is bounded outwardly by the Island of Reil, but which consists of bundles of association

[1] *Dictionary of Terms dealing with Disorders of Speech, op. cit.,* p. 5.

fibres, to and from various parts of the cortex and spinal cord, the lesion is subcortical, and the intellect is not lost.

Déjerine took issue with Marie, holding that motor, visual and auditory defects in speech were evoked by lesions of the frontal, angular and supramarginal gyri, respectively.[1]

Eliasberg holds that aphasia is a unitary disturbance involving impairment of the capacity for speech-expression and speech-comprehension. His methods are: (A) the Direct, with observation of the speech disorder in the individual, including experimental analysis of self-observation on the part of the patient; and (B) the Indirect, involving biological study, observation from the standpoint of anatomy and pathology, and comparison with other aphasias and speech disturbances; (C) the Fundamentally Critical Method in which the disturbance of the intellect is studied as a whole. This involves the belief that pure motor and sensory aphasias do not exist, but that there are mixed forms which overlap in symptomatology and in manifestation of speech and allied expressive activities.[2]

Hughlings-Jackson observed that the majority of aphasics were not aphasic in all situations. If the mechanistic theories of aphasia held, there would always be an inability to read, write, speak or perform the particular function involved in the disability. But Jackson found that it was sometimes present, while at other times the patient could react quite normally in a given speech situation. He also observed that when the patient's speech involved that which was personal or essential to himself, he could answer, but when it involved an artificial situation, such as naming an object, or giving abstract answers, the patient was unable to reply. He responded in *real* situations, but was unable to respond in

[1] Head, H., *Aphasia*, Vol. I, p. 76.

[2] Eliasberg, " Die Schwierigkeit intellektueller Vorgänge, ihre Psychologie, Psychopathologie und ihre Bedeutung für die Intelligenz und Demenzforschung ", Schweiz, *Arch. f. Neurol.*, 1923, Bd. 12.

*Ibid., D. Klin. Beste Wochenschr.*, 1922.

Fröschels, E., *Psychological Elements in Speech*, 1932, pp. 40–6.

any " theoretical " situation. Jackson further distinguished three types of language : (A) common language, (B) emotional language, and (C) intellectual language. He found that the majority of aphasic cases involved the intellectual or third form. One and two might remain intact.[1]

Jackson maintained that it was in the associative realm that most of the aphasic disturbances were found, and that it was difficult to demonstrate a pure sensory or motor aphasia. His findings gave new meaning to the phenomena of the aphasias. It was in the intellectual function that he found most of the aphasics were unable to respond normally. The common language was present, and the emotional-personal language remained, but the more abstract or intellectual language, or that most recently developed in the process of evolution, was the first to suffer, and was the form of speech or expression which suffered the most marked impairment in aphasic attacks.

Jackson's work was followed by that of Head and by the Dutch worker Van Woerkom, by the German psychologist Gelb and by Goldstein, a neurologist. In substance they found that we have a loss of function or reduction in cortical activity at times, but that there is not always a loss of speech and of related activities. They attempted therefore to find in what ways there might be manifestations of symptoms during such cortical reduction, since the speech itself was not always involved. Von Woerkom found that accountants, for instance, were able to perform complicated mathematical problems during attacks of aphasia, but they failed to identify the meanings of isolated numbers. While they could respond in *concrete* situations, they lost the *abstract* meanings of the numbers.

Goldstein held that analysis and treatment of the patient were not to be recommended, when they added to the patient's mental disturbance. He believed that emphasis should be placed upon the changing environ-

---

[1] Head, H., *Aphasia*, Vol. I, pp. 30–53.
   *Ibid.*, *Brain*, 38, 1915, pp. 80–1.

ment for the patient, so that he might respond to simpler conditions of living, which he could understand, and to which he could react normally. He felt that *reality* should be changed for the patient. That is, the environment was to be simplified, rather than to force the patient to remain in a too complex environment, or force him into a new environment where new adjustments would have to be made.

Continuing along the lines suggested by Jackson and Head, Franz has carried researches on dysphasia still further. He regards it as a disability in the formation of associations, explanations of which do not fit into any of the old, neurological classifications of the earlier investigators. He finds that only in a general way is he able to classify aphasics after the divisions of Head, either in living subjects or in post-mortem examination. He finds that the disturbance is more distributed than localized, and that aphasia is characterized by dissociation of ideas, but that *forms* of association *very similar* to those which are lost, remain intact and may be aroused by the same process as that which is intended to arouse the " lost " material. This tends to discredit the theory of " lesion " in that particular speech process in which the " lost " material is stored, and is one of the most important contributions yet made to our study of this subject. According to Franz and other neurologists, it is unsafe to assume that there is a " lead " exercised by one side of the brain over and above that exercised by the other. Assumptions made by those following the lead of Broca, have tended to assume uncritically the fact of such a dominance, and the neurological factors necessary for establishing the theory unquestionably need to be established by other investigators.

One of the important pieces of research undertaken in this connection is that of Travis and Orton,[1] whose

[1] Orton, S. T., " Training the Left Handed ", *Hygeia*, 5, Sept. 1927, pp. 451–4.
*Ibid.* w. Travis, " Studies in Stuttering ", *Arch. Neurol. and Psychiat.*, Nov. 1927, pp. 671–2.

findings are in accordance with the theory of cerebral dominance. They give considerable evidence as to the probability of a "right cerebral lead" for left-handed individuals, and of a "left cerebral lead" for right-handed persons. Until further researches have been offered to substantiate these findings, the question is still undetermined.

While brain destruction is associated with losses of speech and difficulty in forming associations in many organic diseases, we find in dealing with the aphasic, according to Franz, that it is to the *associative* losses that we need to attend. Speech therapy is more successful, when we attempt speech rehabilitation in connection with the associative processes, as illustrated by the use of the various association tests employed by Franz in his re-education programme for aphasics. Classification and localization tend to lead only to confusion, and to neurological and grammatical distinctions which are not yet in accordance with any well-substantiated findings, either on a neurological or on a psychological basis. The present apparent contradictions in terminology may be very well explained on the basis of the theory of Associative Losses, and failure to re-establish connections in the word memory processes, even though other words closely associated with them may be recalled. At what point or in what zones the actual blocking occurs, and how it occurs or why, is still a matter of conjecture, the proof for which may eventually be forthcoming, on the basis of researches being now carried on in various laboratories.

We may find that a strict localization of any type is impossible due to the diffuse nature of the disturbance, and to variations in speech reactions at different times. The "verbal" losses of one type may be replaced by others which are to all intents and purposes of the same significance or importance as the words which are lost. When one response of the "nominal" type disappears, many others often remain, and the associative processes function so that the patient may easily give an extensive list of words suggested by the one which is lost, *even though the particular word itself* cannot be recalled or reproduced. This failure in reproduction is similar to that which occurs in retrograde amnesia, and in normal inability to form associations under stress and strain, as in an important examination, written or oral.

The " syntactical aphasia " of Head [1] also varies from time to time, according to Franz, and the type of " jargon speech " or grammatical disturbance present may be very marked at one time, while speech may appear normal or only slightly disturbed, at other times. The child, in learning to talk, passes through such a process, and the adult who is trying to acquire a new language. The disturbances in forming associations, in fixation, recognition and recall are very similar to those occurring in dysphasia, as one must think almost simultaneously in two languages, and be able to form immediately the necessary connections between them, even though the word-order is not the same, and therefore even the expression of ideas must be inverted, or transposed. This is a much more complicated and difficult process than we realize.

" Semantic " defects also show general and varying losses of power of association, rather than specific and invariable losses. They are not always of the same type, but vary with the nature of the stimulus, and with the mental and physical condition of the patient.

The historical classification of aphasia implies that the groups are mutually exclusive, whereas according to recent investigations, they are usually overlapping. Franz defines aphasia as a loss of associative ability and of some kinds of reduction in cortical or subcortical activity, such as in verbalizing, naming, word-arrangement, ideo-motor processes, often with the retention of other kinds (as in writing). He would direct attention to the relearning, reacquisition or re-formation of associations.[2]

Let us consider some of the ways in which the formation of associations may be blocked or impeded before they

---

[1] Head, *Aphasia*, II, pp. vii–xxiv.

[2] Franz, S. I., " The Relations of Aphasia ", *Jour. of Gen. Psychol.*, 1930, III, 401–11.

arouse the specific neural energy necessary for their discharge over the peripheral nervous tracts, which lead to the speech organs. In the following schematic diagram

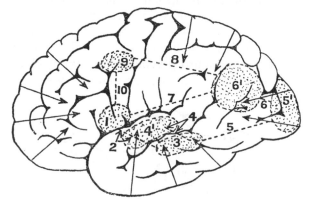

FIG. 1. LEFT CEREBRAL HEMISPHERE

Schematic diagram showing the language zones and connecting pathways, the numerals indicating the speech zones or connections where interference in the transmission of various types of speech impulses may occur.

1. Emissive or motor speech area.
2. Connection between emissive speech area and audito-sensory area.
3. Auditory-perceptual area.
4. Connection between auditory-sensory and auditory-perceptual area.
$4^1$. Auditory-sensory area.
5. Connection between the audito-psychic area and the visuo-sensory area.
$5^1$. Visual-sensory area.
6. Connection between the visual-sensory and visual-psychic areas.
$6^1$. Visual-psychic or perceptual area.
7. Connection between the visual-sensory and visual-psychic areas and the emissive speech area.
8. Connection between the visual-sensory and visual-psychic areas and the graphic or writing centre.
9. Graphic or writing area.
10. Connection between the graphic area and the emissive speech area.

NOTE.—Arrows show how impulses may be transmitted from the higher sensory and motor cortical areas, where it is assumed that associations are formed, connected with the higher learning processes, these psychic "influences" re-enforcing, inhibiting or directing the speech activity.

(Fig. 1) we observe that blocking may occur in any one of a number of different language "zones", or in the transmission of visual, auditory or motor speech impulses from one part of the brain to another. The blocking may be cortical or subcortical, and may involve (1) some part of the emissive speech area, or (2) association fibres between the emissive speech area and the audito-sensory area for the reception of speech sounds, in the temporal lobe ; (3) it may involve the area for sound analysis in the audito-sensory zone ; (4) the difficulty may be in transmission between the audito-sensory and audito-perceptual (audito-psychic) zone ; (5) blocking may occur between the audito-psychic and the visuo-sensory,

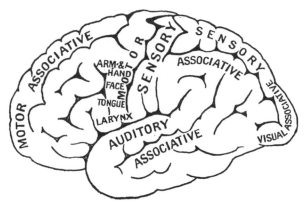

FIG. 2.

Diagram showing integration of the motor and sensory associative areas of the left cerebral hemisphere during speech activity.

or (6) visuo-psychic areas, or (7) the interference may occur between the visual-language-sensory or psychic zones and the speech emissive area ; or (8) between the visual-sensory or psychic and the graphic or writing zone. Finally, in the transmission of a speech impulse, blocking may occur at any one of a number of places not specified in such a schematic representation, but there may be subcortical dissociation or loss of power of formation of associations occurring between any of the above named zones which are concerned with the higher intellectual processes.

That both hemispheres function in the formation of

NOTE.—Figs. 1 and 2 are from drawings made by Dr. C. L. Hawk.

associations and in inner speech is the present opinion of leading neurologists, but that one hemisphere tends to exert a " lead " over the other in controlling the external speech process, or overt language, seems to be in accordance with experimental evidence.  In the right-handed person, according to this theory, the left and right hemispheres function in speech understanding or in internal speech, which requires less of a motor excitation than does external speech.  For external speech the highest centres of the brain are called into action, and in the right-handed person the necessary control seems to be exercised by the third frontal convolution of the left brain, the so-called Broca's area.  For the left-handed person just the reverse is true, according to this supposition. Disturbances of speech of the dysphasia type should be interpreted as primarily associative disturbances, which are diffuse and which may involve any part of the language zones, in the frontal, temporal or occipital lobes, cortical or subcortical or both, and which often may not be due to a distinctly localized or anatomically demonstrable lesion.

Briefly, the common historical classification of aphasia forming the basis of the older theories is as follows :—

1. Agraphia ;  motor aphasia, characterized by loss of writing.

2. Alexia ;  visual-sensory aphasia, characterized by loss of power to comprehend written (or printed) words, due to lesions within the visual centre for words (word-blindness).

3. Articulatory aphasia, or motor, characterized by loss of power to pronounce words or to initiate speech correctly.

4. Auditory aphasia or word-deafness ;  auditory-sensory aphasia, characterized by loss of power to repeat words heard, or to write from dictation, or to understand words spoken.

5. Mixed aphasia ;  characterized by such disorders as agrammaphasia, syntactical aphasia, word-salad speech, groping speech, repetitious speech or paraphasia.

L

6. Total aphasia, characterized by complete loss of speech, in which there are both sensory and motor disturbances.

A revised classification calls for a restatement of Dysphasias as follows : Dysphasia may be of an organic or functional type, cortical or subcortical in origin, characterized by loss of power of association or disintegration between any of the various language zones and the peripheral speech mechanism, and involving any combination of the following types :—

1. Dysgraphia ; disturbances in writing.
2. Dyslexia, visuo-sensory or visuo-psychic disturbances ; word-blindness.
3. Articulatory motor dysphasia ; emissive speech.
4. Audito-sensory or audito-psychic dysphasia (cortical or subcortical) ; word-deafness.
5. Mixed dysphasias, motor, sensory and associational ; integrative process.
6. Aphasia.

*Causes.*—One of the most frequent causes of organic aphasia is hemorrhage of the mid-cerebral artery. The prognosis in the case of apoplexy is not good. Dysphasia of the organic type follows cerebral lesions, also, and may be due to brain injury, brain disease or to traumatic shocks. Temporary or permanent disorders of association are common, and there is usually some permanent reduction in cortical activity, following an attack of dysphasia. There is a diffuse, general impairment of ideational levels, manifested by disturbances in associative thinking and loss of integration in those cortical or subcortical functions, the integrity of which is necessary for the possession of normal speech.

Dysphasia of the functional or associative type is manifested by disturbances in associative thinking, and is a psychic phenomenon which may not be accounted for on the basis of any disease, lesion or other demonstrable organic anomaly. The customary speech and related activities as in reading, writing, arousal of auditory or visual word-memories, musical memories, or mathematical symbols, may be impaired or lost. The speech disturbance may be manifested by (1) word mutilation; (2) word reduction; (3) paraphasia; (4) inability to recall words associated with the higher intellectual processes, although words having emotional significance may be retained; (5) inability to repeat after another person dictated words; (6) complete or partial loss of expression in the form of spontaneous speech; (7) occurrence of repetitious speech without comprehension of meaning; (8) disturbances in association and comprehension of ideas involving any of the language processes, such as the audito-sensory or visuo-sensory and psychic language areas; (9) various forms of dysphasia involving any of the internal ideational levels and the external speech processes, and varying from time to time in their manifestations.

Improvement depends upon the patient's organic condition, and upon nature of the destruction occurring in the cortical region, in brain disease in which there are cerebral lesions. In forms of dysphasia in which there is no organic lesion, improvement depends upon the patient's power to re-form associations between words, and to regain his " intellectual " speech, as well as to retain his common, emotional language.[1]

[1] For speech re-education, see Franz Aphasia testing material.

# Part II

## STATISTICAL STUDIES

OF

## THE SPEECH OF 3000 COLLEGE WOMEN

AND OF

## PUBLIC SCHOOL GROUPS

# CHAPTER VIII

## ANALYSIS OF SPEECH DATA SHEET FOR 412 COLLEGE AND PUBLIC SCHOOL STUDENTS

1. Mount Holyoke Corrective Speech Group, Fall of 1931 . . . . . . . . 25 Students
2. Mount Holyoke College Control Group of . 259 ,,
   (Entering students, Fall of 1931, including all girls not held for speech correction)
3. Hunter College Corrective Group . . . 25 ,,
4. Hunter College Control Group . . . 25 ,,
5. San Francisco Corrective Group . . . 22 ,,
6. Chicago Corrective Group . . . . 18 ,,
7. Chicago Control Group . . . . . 12 ,,
8. Tampa Class in Public Speaking . . . 12 ,,
9. London Corrective Group . . . . 14 ,,

Total . 412 ,,

IN addition to the Thurstone Personality Schedule a speech data sheet devised by the writer was given at Mount Holyoke College in the Fall of 1931 as a part of the speech tests which are given to all entering students. The purpose of this data sheet was to secure more information concerning the student than is usually given on college entrance papers, and the questions asked were so arranged that the instructor might ascertain very quickly the student's position in the family, her former training in speech, degree of excellence in speech, disorders or difficulty in speech, and lessons or treatments received for same. A subjective estimate of the student's own vocal reactions included auditory responses to vocalizations of various types, speech discriminative ability, personality judgments based on speech, characteristics of the " pleasantest voices " heard either in one's social group, or among public speakers or radio entertainers. The effect of speech upon personality, in case of a speech handicap, and the qualities of leadership developed in

167

more aggressive students, were also included in the list of questions. Some questions could be answered by *Yes* or *No*, while others could be underlined, or an alternative answer written in the space provided. The student was told that the information contained was to be treated confidentially and that it would be accessible only to members of the departments of speech and psychology.

This questionnaire was given to the entire entering class in the Fall of 1931, consisting of 291 students. The speech *corrective group* (I) was separately summarized and compared with the remaining or *non-corrective* groups making up Groups II, III and IV (*i.e.* those in Freshman required speech classes, those deferred to one of the upper class years, for their speech requirement, and a small group of students excused from speech because of entrance with advanced standing).

The questions or statements to which answers were required, are as follows :—

### SPEECH DATA SHEET
*(This material will be treated confidentially)*

*Directions.*—Some of the following statements may be answered by enclosing in a circle the (Yes) or the (No) ; others may be answered by *underlining* the term which best applies to your own speech situation ; still others may be answered by writing in a short statement in the spaces provided. Please answer *every item* in one of the above-mentioned ways. You will be given plenty of time to complete it, but please work as rapidly as you can.

1. Your name...........................................
2. Age .....................................................
3. Sex (*underline*) M.  F.
4. Own occupation (*underline* or write) student, teacher (or)
   ....................
5. Father's occupation .......................................
6. School last attended.......................................
7. Home address.............................................
8. { Local address...........................................
   { Phone number ........................................
9. Place of birth ...........................................
10. Draw a line after the correct number to indicate the number of children in your family, and underline your position in it. For example (1 2 3 4 5/6 7 8 9 10). This means that the underlined is the first-born or eldest, and that there

are five children in the family. (*Answer here*) 1 2 3 4 5 6 7 8 9 10. How many years are there between you and your next oldest brother or sister ?....................
How many years between you and the next youngest brother or sister ?....................

11. Are you well satisfied with your speech as it is ? (*underline*) Yes. No.

12. In what way, if any, would you like to improve it ? ........ ....................

13. Do you sing ? (*underline*) Yes. No.

14. Debate ? Yes. No.

15. Have you taken part in more than one play ? Yes. No.

16. Do you like to talk ? Yes. No.

17. Have you had any special training in speech ? Yes. No.

18. Of what kind ? ....................

19. Have you ever had lessons or treatment for the correction of speech difficulty, loss of voice, lisping or stuttering, etc. ? Yes. No.

20. Explain which of the above, by underlining one, or writing in ....................

21. Where or from whom have you received such corrective treatment, if any ? ....................

22. For how long continued ? ....................

23. Can you carry a tune easily ? Yes. No.

24. Play a musical instrument ? Yes. No....................

25. Do you seem to hear certain kinds of tones better than others ? Yes. No.

26. Do you ever lose your voice completely ? Yes. No.

27. Do you usually notice when a person is singing or playing off-key ? Yes. No.

28. Are you quick to notice differences in people's voices ? Yes. No.

29. Differences in accent and pronunciation ? Yes. No.

30. Can you imitate accents or unusual speech and dialect, quite readily ? Yes. No.

31. What peculiarities in the voices of people do you notice most easily ? .................... (write in or *underline* any of the following) :  Sound of voice, accent, pronunciation, dialect, personality of the speaker.

32. Which of the following seems easiest for you ?  Conversation, reading poetry or prose, argumentation, talking in a group, talking to one person, talking to men, talking to women, taking part in a play, talking to yourself when alone ? (Write in own answer, or *underline* above)..............

33. Are you accustomed to judge people more by the way they speak, the way they dress, or the way they look in general ? (*underline*)

34. What are you able to tell about a person, by his voice or speech ? .................... If you find this difficult, try to recall the voice of some prominent person whom you have recently heard speaking in public or over the radio, and tell what qualities that particular voice suggested to you ? ....................

35. If you cannot recall any such speech, think of some acquaintance of yours with well-marked vocal characteristics, pleasant or otherwise, and use this voice to help you answer the above question. ...................

36. Give several characteristics of the pleasantest voice you know....................

37. Were you influenced more by the voice, appearance, or by the personality of the person recalled, in making your list of characteristics of " the pleasantest voice " ?..............

38. What do you consider to be the chief characteristics of the cultured speech of the college man or woman ? (Write in here, or *underline* any of the following)...............
    well-modulated voice, smooth utterance, clearness in speech, intelligibility, good vocal quality, low pitch, moderate rate in speech, medium loudness (not soft, and not over-boisterous tones), good variety in intonation, matter-of-fact tones, " plain speech ", decisive, crisp utterance, animated tones (etc.)....................

39. Did you ever leave school because of your speech ? Yes. No.

40. Is your own speech (*underline*) good, bad, average (or fair) ?

41. Have you a pleasing voice ? Yes. No.

42. Is your accent and pronunciation like that of most of your friends ? Yes. No.

43. If not, how does it differ ?...................

44. Are you a leader in your social group ? Yes. No.

45. Do you usually prefer to have someone else take the initiative ? Yes. No.

46. Have you ever felt inferior because of poor speech or personality ? (*Underline* the appropriate one, in the above statement.) Yes. No.

47. Did you ever have any severe frights or shocks in childhood which in any way explain a possible speech difficulty, since ? Yes. No.

48. Explain in a brief statement.............................
    ...........................................
    Add below anything else which you think might be important in interpreting this record.
    ............................................ ..
    ............................................

The data sheet was also given to 25 students in a speech correction group at Hunter College, New York, and to 25 students in artistic speech courses, the latter serving as a control group.[1] For purposes of comparison and in order to ascertain some of the differences in character of answers given by a college group as compared with outside groups of high school or college age, the same

[1] Data secured by Miss Jane B. Taylor, Department of Speech, Hunter College.

questionnaire was given to all the students in a high school speech corrective group in San Francisco,[1] to two groups in a Chicago Technical High School,[2] to a group in a class in public speaking in Tampa, Florida,[3] and to a hospital speech-clinic group in London.[4]

The age and sex distribution for the different groups was as follows: Table I; *Questions 2 and 3.*

### TABLE I

TITLE OF GROUP

| Mount Holyoke Groups | | Hunter College Group | San Francisco Group | | Chicago Group | | Tampa Group | | London Group | |
|---|---|---|---|---|---|---|---|---|---|---|
| | F * | F | F | M | F | M | F | M | F | M |
| Corrective . | 25 | 25 | 5 | 17 | — | 30 | 6 | 6 | 2 | 12 |
| Control . | 259 | 25 | — | — | — | — | — | — | — | — |
| Totals | 284 | 50 | 22 | | 30 | | 12 | | 14 | |

MEDIAN AGE

| Mount Holyoke Groups | Hunter College Group, | San Francisco Group | Chicago Group | Tampa Group | London Group |
|---|---|---|---|---|---|
| Corrective . 18 | 18 | 14 | 18 | 19½ | 17 |
| Control . 17 | 18 | — | 17 | — | — |
| Median for College Groups = 18 | | | Median for all other groups = 17 | | |

\* *Key* : F=Female.    M=Male.

In the Tampa and San Francisco classes the questions were given to students in only one class, and not checked against any control group. It will be seen that the students in both the Chicago and Mount Holyoke control groups above have a slight age advantage over the corrective groups in both instances, the girls in Mount Holyoke corrective group and the boys in the Chicago Technical High School group in speech correction averaging one year older than the non-correctives in both institutions. The median age for the matched groups at Hunter College, corrective and control, is the same.

[1] Miss Edna Cotrel.
[3] E. K. Hartzell.
[2] Miss Martha Dwyer.
[4] Miss E. Kingdon Ward.

*Questions 4 and 5.—Own Occupation ; Parents' Occupation*

*Own Occupation.*[1]—In all except the London corrective and the Tampa group the subjects were students in college or in public school. The Tampa and London groups contained adults from occupational groups I and III as follows :—

|  | Tampa Group | London Group |
|---|---|---|
| Group I. Professional . . . . . . . | 7 | 7 |
| Group II. Semi-professional (managers, proprietors, etc.) . . . . . . . . . | — | — |
| Group III. Skilled labourers (clerks, salesmen, mechanics, retailers) . . . . . . | 5 | 6 |
| Group IV. Semi-skilled labourers (farmers, bakers, painters, chauffeurs, barbers, waiters, etc.) . | — | — |
| Group V. Common labourer or unskilled worker . | — | I |
| Total . . | 12 | 14 |

*Occupation of Parents.*—The occupation of parents was given by 249 out of 259 Mount Holyoke girls in the control group, and by 25 girls in the speech corrective group.

| OCCUPATIONAL GROUPING | CORRECTIVE GROUPS | | CONTROL GROUPS | |
|---|---|---|---|---|
|  | Mount Holyoke | Hunter College* | Mount Holyoke | Hunter College* |
|  | Per cent. of those in this ...... group | | Per cent. in group | |
| I. Professional . . | 52 | 5 | 41·1 | 4 |
| II. Semi-professional : |  |  |  |  |
|     Type A . . . | 24 | 45 | 34·1 | 13 |
|     Type B . . . | 20 | 25 | 19·6 | 13 |
| III. Skilled occupational | 4 | 25 | 2 | 31 |
| IV. Semi-skilled level . | — | — | — | 31 |
| V. Unskilled . . | — | — | — | 8 |

* Based on 34 parents whose occupations were given, in Hunter groups, ...... 16 parents deceased.

[1] Fryer, D., *School and Society*, Vol. XVI, No. 401, pp. 273–277, Sept. 1922.

Terman, *Genetic Studies of Genius*, Vol. I, p. 64.

Taussig's *Five Point Scale*, ibid., Vol. I, pp. 63–64.

This indicates that a larger percentage of Mount Holyoke girls in the corrective group come from a superior professional, cultural background than do the girls who are not held for speech corrective work. This is rather surprising, and seems to imply that homes of culture are not always safeguards against the appearance of speech defects in members of such families. The highest percentage of the girls in the control group come from families found in Group II, Types A and B, the first representing a slightly higher gradation than the second within this group. A smaller percentage of girls in the corrective group come from this type of background. Twice as many (4 per cent.) of the corrective group appear in the Group III (skilled occupational level) as in the control group (2 per cent.). Groups IV and V, semi-skilled and unskilled, are not represented in either group.

The occupational background for Hunter College groups varies from that given for the Mount Holyoke groups, as in the latter the highest percentage in the corrective group represents professional Group I. In the Hunter College corrective group we find the largest number of students come from parental background Group II, semi-professional, while in the control group an equal number come from Groups III and IV (skilled occupational level and semi-skilled). In the corrective group a larger percentage come from Type A (45 per cent.) and somewhat less (25 per cent.) in Type B, making a total of 70 per cent. coming from Group II. In the control group we find an equal number representing Type A and Type B at Hunter College, there being a slight distinction made between these two in Fryer's analysis of occupational levels. There is a total of 26 per cent. The largest number in the Hunter control group represent Groups III and IV (31 per cent. each, or a total of 62 per cent. in all).

Although there are fewer representing the professional group, in the latter table, it is interesting to note that the corrective represents a higher group than found in the table for the control group, and this agrees with the Mount Holyoke findings, in that a higher occupational level was represented in the corrective group, than in the control group, even though the particular groups represented differed in the two colleges.

Mount Holyoke Corrective Group　　Highest percentage from Group I
Mount Holyoke Control Group　　　Highest percentage from Group II
Hunter College Corrective Group　　Highest percentage from Group II
Hunter College Control Group　　　Highest percentage equally divided
　　　　　　　　　　　　　　　　between Groups III and IV.

This again is somewhat in accordance with our findings based on the study in Thurstone's Personality Schedule for the Mount Holyoke Group, that speech defects in college students are more often a matter of adjustment, or due to neurotic factors, than to scholarship, native aptitude, or family status. In the well-adjusted speech groups in both colleges we find that the background has less to do with the matter of speech-defect than we might suppose, as judging from opinion and hearsay. Occupational groups may differ widely in groups from different colleges, but the significant thing here seems to be that the corrective groups in both cases actually come from a supposedly better environment than the control or non-corrective groups as a whole in both institutions.

The occupational levels represented by the public school group are as follows :—

| | San Francisco Group | Chicago Groups | | Tampa Group | London Group |
|---|---|---|---|---|---|
| | | Corrective | Control | | |
| Group I. Professional . . | 2 | — | — | 1 | — |
| Group II. Semi-professional . | — | 1 | — | 4 | — |
| Group III. Skilled labour . | 13 | 8 | 4 | 1 | 10 |
| Group IV. Semi-skilled labour | 5 | 6 | 5 | 3 | 4 |
| Group V. Unskilled labour . | 2 | 3 | 3 [1] | — | 0 |
| Totals . . | 22 | 18 | 12 | 9 | 14 |
| Not stated . . . . | — | — | — | 3 | — |

At Mount Holyoke College we found that the occupational backgrounds of girls, both the controls and the correctives, were largely from Groups I and II as given

[1] Unemployed.

above.    In the Hunter College and the public school groups we find a different occupational status, as the majority in these groups come from occupational groups II, III and IV.

In the Chicago analysis we find that an equal number of those in the corrective-speech group and in the control group come from Group V (unskilled labour).    The background for the largest number of the corrective groups from the public schools as represented in the groups from Chicago, San Francisco and London represent Group III (skilled labour group).    The majority of the adult Tampa Public Speaking Class come from Group II (semi-professional).    While the number of students represented is too small for us to draw any sweeping conclusions, it seems evident that nearly all of those represented, other than the Tampa group, are from occupational levels III and IV, while the Mount Holyoke and Hunter College groups, corrective and non-corrective, represent largely occupational groups I and II or III.    A small number of the Mount Holyoke group come from occupational group III, but none from Groups IV and V.    Teachers of speech correction in different environments are dealing with offspring from very different social backgrounds as shown by comparison of groups in speech correction in the public schools and in colleges or universities.    This difference may be significant in regard to corrective measures applied and permanent results gained with these groups.    It may require a different type of speech therapy.

*Question* 10.—*Position in Family*

In the Mount Holyoke corrective group 18 were first-born or eldest, 6 were second-born, 1 was third in the family.    In the control group by far the greatest number were eldest or first-born, the next largest being second-born.    In no case were there more than eight children in a family.    In the corrective group, about one-third were only children, whereas 67 out of the control group of 259, or about one-quarter, were only children.    The median number of years between the student and older siblings was 2 years for the Mount Holyoke corrective group, and 3 years for the control group. The median number of years between the student and younger siblings was 2½ years in the corrective group, and 3 years in the

TABLE II

| Position in Family | 1st | 2nd | 3rd | 4th | 5th | 6th | 7th | 8th | 9th | 10th | 11th | 12th |
|---|---|---|---|---|---|---|---|---|---|---|---|---|
| San Francisco group (Median position 2nd or 3rd child) | 6 | 5 | 7 | 3 | 1 | — | — | — | — | — | — | — |
| Chicago Groups | | | | | | | | | | | | |
| a. Corrective . | 4 | 5 | 4 | 3 | 2 | — | 1 | — | — | — | — | — |
| b. Control . | 5 | 3 | 1 | 1 | — | — | — | — | — | — | — | — |
| (Median position, 2nd, both groups) | | | | | | | | | | | | |
| Tampa Group . (Median, 2nd) | 1 | 5 | 1 | 3 | — | — | 1 | — | — | — | — | 1 |
| Mount Holyoke Corrective Group . (Median 1st born) | 18 | 6 | 1 | — | — | — | — | — | — | — | — | — |
| Mount Holyoke Control Group (Median 2nd born) | 118 | 90 | 33 | 7 | 6 | 3 | — | 1 | — | — | — | — |
| London Corrective (Median 2nd born) | 4 | 7 | 2 | — | 1 | — | — | — | — | — | — | — |

As to " only children " the following results were tabulated :

| | |
|---|---|
| San Francisco Group (Corrective) . . | 3 |
| Chicago Corrective Group . . . | 0 |
| Chicago Control Group . . . | 2 |
| Tampa Group (public speaking) . . | 2 |
| Mount Holyoke Corrective Group . . | 9 (out of 25) |
| Mount Holyoke Control Group . . | 67 (out of 259) |
| London Corrective Group . . . | 1 |

control group. This seems to bear out the findings of Thurstone that position in family is less significant in the development of neurotic tendencies than is generally believed, as the differences in position in families are slight as between the corrective and the control groups.[1]

In the Hunter College corrective group five were first-

[1] Thurstone, L. L., " Neurotic Inventory," A. Jour. of Soc. Psychol., I, 1930, pp. 25–6.

born and nine were second-born, there being a smaller number occupying other positions in the family group. In the control group there were an equal number (six of each) who were first-born and second-born, with a few occupying other positions in the family. There were six " only children " in the Hunter College control group, and two " only children " in the corrective group. The median position in both of the Hunter College groups was second-born. This agrees with the findings for Mount Holyoke groups, in which it seems that position in the family is less important than has been believed. The median number of years between the student and older or younger siblings was two years in both Hunter College groups. There were more " only children " in the control than in the corrective group.

The distribution of students as to locality was as follows for the Mount Holyoke groups. The Hunter College and the public school groups were local pupils living in the cities studied.

MOUNT HOLYOKE GROUPS

| | France | N.Y. | N.J. | Mass. | Conn. | R.I. | Ill. | Neb. | Ky. | Pa. |
|---|---|---|---|---|---|---|---|---|---|---|
| A. Corrective Group . | 1 | 10 | 5 | 3 | 1 | 1 | 1 | 1 | 1 | — |
| B. Control Group . | — | 82 | 32 | 47 | 25 | 7 | 6 | — | 1 | 23 |

In both of the above groups the largest number come from New York State, this being the State having the largest representation in the class as a whole in the fall of 1931. In the corrective group New Jersey and Massachusetts stood second and third in relation to numbers, while in the control group the order is just reversed and Connecticut stands in fourth place. Pennsylvania stands fifth in the control group, but is not represented in the corrective group. All other States having a comparatively slight representation, are omitted from the table. Twenty-four States were represented in the class and there is no

M

significant difference in locale as between the corrective
and control groups as given above.

*Question 11.—Are you well satisfied with your speech as it is ?*

| Answers | Yes | No | Unan-swered | Fairly so |
|---|---|---|---|---|
| Mount Holyoke Corrective Group | 6 | 18 | 1 | — |
| Mount Holyoke Control Group . | 62 | 191 | 5 | 1 |
| Hunter College Corrective Group | 1 | 23 | 1 | — |
| Hunter College Control Group . | 4 | 21 | — | — |
| San Francisco Group (Corrective) | 4 | 18 | — | — |
| Chicago Corrective Group . . | 3 | 15 | — | — |
| Chicago Control Group . . | 7 | 5 | — | — |
| Tampa Public Speaking Group . | 1 | 11 | — | — |
| London Corrective Group . . | 1 | 12 | 1 | — |

About one-third of the students in both Mount Holyoke
groups expressed themselves as dissatisfied with their
speech. Most of the Hunter corrective group and one-
fifth of the control group answered in the affirmative.
In the public school groups we find that both the San
Francisco and Chicago corrective groups expressed themselves as critical of their speech, as did also the majority
of the members of the Tampa group. This should prove
a helpful point in training, as it indicates a readiness to
undertake measures for voice improvement.

*Question 12.—In what way, if any, would you like to
improve it ? (Speech)*

The Mount Holyoke group of correctives answered this
most frequently by using the following descriptive terms:—

| | |
|---|---|
| Enunciation | Poise |
| Vocal quality | Eliminate lisping |
| Slower speech | Eliminate stuttering |
| Distinctness | Increase volume of tone |

The Mount Holyoke control group answered most
frequently as follows :—

| | | |
|---|---|---|
| Enunciation | Articulation | Vocabulary |
| Voice and tone (quality) | Clearness | Tone projection |
| | Diction | Pronunciation |
| Slower speech | Volume | Lower pitch |
| Distinctness | Fluency | |

Summarizing the answers given by the city school groups, including the San Francisco, Chicago and Tampa groups, we find the following were listed most frequently :—

| | | |
|---|---|---|
| Distinctness | Effective utterance | Stuttering |
| Conversational power | Expression | Lisping |
| Overcome nasality | Improve vocabulary | Tonal quality |
| Learn to debate | Learn to speak in public | Slower speech |
| Correct speech | Smoothness | Speak plainly |
| Enunciation | | |

The Hunter College corrective group answered most frequently with these terms :—

Speech defect    Voice and diction    Improve speech generally

The control group answered chiefly as follows :—

| | | | |
|---|---|---|---|
| Voice | Quality | Generally | Vocabulary |
| Accent | Pronunciation | | |

*Question 13.—Do you sing ?*

| Answers | Yes | No | Some | Unans. |
|---|---|---|---|---|
| Mount Holyoke Corrective Group | 12 | 13 | — | — |
| Mount Holyoke Control Group  . | 127 | 126 | 1 | 5 |
| Hunter College Corrective Group | 16 | 9 | — | — |
| Hunter College Control Group   . | 12 | 12 | — | — |
| San Francisco Group (Corrective) | 17 | 5 | — | — |
| Chicago Corrective Group .    . | 13 | 5 | — | — |
| Chicago Control Group    .    . | 8 | 4 | — | — |
| Tampa Public Speaking Group  . | 7 | 4 | — | 1 |
| London Corrective Group .    . | 7 | 6 | — | — |

The corrective group, in proportion to its size, shows no fewer students who are interested in singing than does the control group. Half of the students in both groups at Mount Holyoke answered in the negative and half in the affirmative, which seems to indicate that in these particular groups at least, there is no difference in amount of vocal training received. More girls from the corrective group answered this question in the affirmative. Answers from the control group are half in the affirmative and half in the negative, both at Mount Holyoke and at Hunter College. In the San Francisco and Chicago corrective groups more than twice as many students report themselves as interested in singing, than report in the negative. This might seem significant, were it not also the case that the next two groups, the Chicago control group and the Tampa public speaking group answer in the affirmative in larger numbers than in the negative. Possibly the factor of public school training in music for all students explains the answers obtained here, and it is fairer to assume that the factor of general musical training, rather than special musical interest or attempts at compensation for ineffective speech, are the explanations for these answers, rather than to assume that more students sing or do not sing, in any of the above groups, on the basis of compensation for speech inadequacy.

### Question 14.—*Do you debate ?*

| Answers | Yes | No | Unans. | Occasionally |
|---|---|---|---|---|
| Mount Holyoke Corrective Group | 5 | 20 | — | — |
| Mount Holyoke Control Group . | 44 | 198 | 6 | 2 |
| Hunter College Corrective Group | 9 | 16 | — | — |
| Hunter College Control Group . | 3 | 22 | — | — |
| San Francisco Group . . | 6 | 16 | — | — |
| Chicago Corrective Group . . | 6 | 12 | — | — |
| Chicago Control Group . . | 5 | 6 | 1 | — |
| Tampa Public Speaking Group . | 3 | 9 | — | — |
| London Corrective Group . . | 3 | 9 | — | — |

It is rather surprising to find that only about one-fourth of both the Mount Holyoke corrective and control groups are familiar with debating from personal participation. One-half of the Hunter College corrective group and one-seventh of the control group have participated in debate. About one-third of the San Francisco and the Chicago corrective groups have engaged in debate ; about one-fourth of the Tampa group ; the Chicago control group shows about an equal number who do or do not debate.

### Question 15.—*Have you taken part in more than one play ?*

| Answers | Yes | No | Unans. |
|---|---|---|---|
| Mount Holyoke Corrective Group . . | 19 | 6 | — |
| Mount Holyoke Control Group . . | 179 | 78 | 2 |
| Hunter College Corrective Group . . | 18 | 7 | — |
| Hunter College Control Group . . | 17 | 7 | — |
| San Francisco Corrective Group . . | 15 | 6 | 1 |
| Chicago Corrective Group . . | 13 | 5 | — |
| Chicago Control Group . . . | 7 | 5 | — |
| Tampa Public Speaking Group . . | 6 | 6 | — |
| London Corrective Group . . . | 5 | 9 | — |

It is significant that in all but the London corrective and the Tampa groups a large number report that they have taken part in plays. The proportion of those in the Mount Holyoke corrective groups who have participated in plays is smaller in proportion to the size of the group than in the control group. Even though participation is, as we should anticipate, facilitated by freedom from speech defects, and students with good speech are usually more readily cast in various roles than are those possessing a speech impediment, the corrective student is often quite as anxious to try-out or to participate, as are his more fluent companions. His attempts at compensation thus bear fruit more often than we should have anticipated, considering his speech difficulty.

*Question 16.—Do you like to talk ?*

| Answers | Yes | No | Some-times | Inform-ally | Unan-swered | Total |
|---|---|---|---|---|---|---|
| Mount    Holyoke    Corrective Group    .    .    .    . | 17 | 8 | — | — | — | 25 |
| Mount Holyoke Control Group | 182 | 67 | 4 | 1 | 2 | 256 |
| Hunter    College    Corrective Group    .    .    .    . | 21 | 4 | — | — | — | 25 |
| Hunter College Control Group | 22 | 2 | — | — | 1 | 25 |
| San Francisco Corrective Group | 19 | 3 | — | — | — | 22 |
| Chicago Corrective Group    . | 13 | 5 | — | — | — | 18 |
| Chicago Control Group .    . | 9 | 3 | — | — | — | 12 |
| Tampa Group    .    .    . | 8 | 4 | — | — | — | 12 |
| London Corrective Group    . | 10 | 3 | — | — | 1 | 14 |

In every instance there was a higher percentage of positive than of negative answers. The highest frequencies were for the Hunter College groups and for the San Francisco corrective group, in which 84 to 88 per cent. of the pupils expressed a liking for self-expression. The next highest frequency was for Chicago control group in which 75 per cent. reported positively, while in the Chicago corrective group a similar number of 72 per cent. reported positively. In the Mount Holyoke control group 71 per cent. of the students answered in the affirmative, while 68 per cent. of the corrective group so reported. In the Tampa group, which corresponds more closely in character to the Mount Holyoke groups, than do the public school groups, we find 66 per cent. reporting in the affirmative. In the London group 71 per cent. report in the affirmative. The only conclusion we may draw from this is, that the speech handicap does not interfere with the desire or ambition to engage in speech as a form of expression, and whatever the speech handicap, the students in the corrective groups in general are quite as desirous of using this outlet for self-expression as are those who are unaware of any such handicap. In the larger groups, such as the Holyoke corrective and control groups, the girls with better speech seem to enjoy self-expression scarcely any more than do those in the speech-corrective group.

It seems to the writer that there is no real desire on the part of these students to inhibit speech responses, and to appear poorly socialized, but that on the contrary they are usually eager to overcome any such tendency, and that this is a point which might be utilized more intelligently by teachers of expression, in planning speech courses or conferences for students with speech handicaps.

*Questions 17–19.—Have you had speech training ? Type ?*
*Have you had lessons for speech correction ?*

| Answers | Yes | No | Type of Training |
|---|---|---|---|
| Mount Holyoke Corrective Group | 9 | 16 | Corrective work (3 students). Public speaking, oratory drama, expression (6 students |
| Mount Holyoke Control Group . | 98 | 161 | Public speaking, expression drama, elocution, phonetics interpretation, oral English debate. |
| Hunter College Corrective Group | 21 | 4 | Phonetics, public speaking interpretation, fundamental speech course. |
| Hunter College Control Group . | 24 | 1 | Phonetics, voice, dramatics public speaking, interpretation. |
| San Francisco Group . . | 4 | 18 | Corrective speech and public speaking. |
| Chicago (Correctives) . . | 18 | — | Corrective speech course (past or present). |
| Chicago (Controls) . . . | 1 | 11 | Expression. |
| Tampa Group. . . . | 4 | 8 | Expression. |
| London Group . . . | 12 | — | Speech Correction. |

Except for the Chicago corrective group, all of whom were receiving corrective aid at the time when the questionnaire was answered, the results seem to indicate that twice as many have received no training in either speech science or speech arts, as have been favoured with such training.    There are indications that students who have had speech training are better speech representatives, however, than those without such training.    The writer compared results of the speech testing at Mount Holyoke in a recent year with results obtained by the staff in speech at Smith College,[1] and in both colleges it was found that the girl from the private school passed the speech tests more easily than did the girl from the public school. Investigations seem to indicate that the private school pays more attention to the individual development, personality and social adjustment in speech, than does the average public school.

Comparing this with the results for Hunter College we find a different situation, however, as here the control group consisted of girls in fundamental speech courses, and all students in the corrective group were required to take the fundamental courses in speech in addition to speech correction.    This explains the higher percentage of positive answers.

SPEECH TRAINING

| Hunter College | . | Corrective Group | . | Yes, 21 | . | No, 4 |
| Hunter College | . | Control Group | . | Yes, 24 | . | No, 1 |

With an increase in the number of courses in speech given in private, public and preparatory schools generally, there has been noticeable for the past three years a slight falling off in the number of girls held for speech correction at Mount Holyoke.    This may be partly as a result of the knowledge that such tests are to be given, and the schools may have stressed this type of preparation more in their candidates, but we believe the slight dropping off is to be explained on the ground of an increase in the number of speech-training courses which are being introduced

[1] Courtesy of Miss Elizabeth Avery, Smith College.

into preparatory schools. We believe this to be a result of an increasing interest in speech and personality development, and in the present emphasis on the individual, in contrast to mass education. This is illustrated by the responses of the Hunter College speech groups on this point.

If, as has been suggested,[1] employers of young business men abroad favour English to American candidates because of the more cultured speech of English University men, then it is not too much to ask of our American Colleges that they require some type of speech preparation as a part of the college training of every candidate for a degree.[1] Not only should this be true of colleges, but of high and preparatory schools generally, as by far the larger number of the young people go out from high school to take up their life work without further opportunity to develop their voice and personality assets, apart from such incidental development as is a part of their regular employment.

During the depression following the World War, it has been shown that the trained man or woman of the skilled or professional classes, has been able to remain employed more readily than the less cultured or less skilled man and woman. Employers demand results, and are insistent upon receiving the best quality of work which can be done, in return for wages expended. Speech culture certainly plays its role in cultural development, self-expression and in other of the higher skills.

*Questions 23–31.—Auditory imagery, pitch discrimination, qualitative differences in voices, etc.*

No. 23. Can you carry a tune ?
No. 24. Can you play a musical instrument ?
No. 25. Do you seem to hear certain notes better than others ?
No. 26. Did you ever suffer from complete loss of voice ?
No. 27. Are you quick to detect off-key notes ?
No. 28. Are you quick to notice differences in people's voices ?

[1] Heltman, H. J., *Speech Manual*, 1932, p. 3.

No. 29. Are you quick to note differences in accent and pronunciation ?

No. 30. Can you do dialect and have you good speech imitative ability ?

No. 31. What peculiarities in voices do you notice most readily ?

### Question 23.—*Ability to carry a tune*

In all of the groups except the Chicago control group and the Hunter College corrective group, responses indicate that at least two-thirds of each group can " carry a tune ".   In the Chicago control and the Hunter corrective group the answers were about evenly divided between positive and negative.

### Question 24.—*Ability to play musical instrument*

In the Mount Holyoke and Hunter College corrective and control groups, the London and San Francisco corrective groups, more than half of the responses were in the affirmative as regards playing a musical instrument. In the Chicago corrective and control groups a larger number reported in the negative, and in the Tampa public speaking group the answers were equally divided between negative and positive.   Differences in cultural backgrounds would seem to explain these differences, rather than any inability to master technique in the corrective as compared with the control groups, as the correctives do not show any less ability in this special skill than do the control groups tested.   Piano, organ, violin, mandolin and saxophone were the instruments most frequently listed.

### Question 25.—*Hearing certain tones better than others*

The question in regard to hearing certain notes better than others was specially designed to find out if, in the corrective group, there might be cases of high-frequency deafness, such as inability to hear *S* sounds clearly. Such cases were then checked up further by giving the Seashore Musical Tests to all members of the speech-corrective group. The results on the latter test are reported in another section.

On this question " *Do you hear certain notes better than others ?* " all except the Tampa group answered mostly with " No ". In the Tampa group the answers were about equally divided between Yes and No. The small number of those in the corrective groups who answered in the affirmative would still be enough to warrant the giving of other tests to determine the acuity of hearing, pitch discrimination and the like, as a basis for the corrective work. In every group there were several individuals who stated that they were not able to distinguish notes equally well. A check by means of the Seashore Musical Test, an articulation test, and an audiometer might enable the examiner to determine whether there exists a high-frequency deafness which makes it impossible for the student to discriminate easily between a correct and an inaccurate $S$ sound. The writer has found that such seems to be the case with a number of students who are in the corrective group because of lisping, and who sometimes cannot hear the difference between the word " sister " as normally spoken, and the substitute sounds in " *thithter* ", as spoken with a lisp.

### Question 26.—Voice

This question in regard to loss of voice seems at first glance to be misplaced, but it is intended primarily to get at the factor of hysterical loss of voice, and deals with the relation between auditory discrimination and emotion, rather than with the physiological inability to phonate.

| Answers (Subject to loss of voice) ? | Yes | No | Unans. | Subject to Laryngitis | | |
|---|---|---|---|---|---|---|
| Mount Holyoke Corrective Group | 4 | 21 | — | — | 1 | — |
| Mount Holyoke Control Group | 20 | 238 | 1 | — | — | — |
| Hunter College Corrective Group | 17 | 8 | — | — | — | — |
| Hunter College Control Group | 5 | 20 | — | — | — | — |
| San Francisco Corrective Group | 3 | 19 | — | — | — | — |
| Chicago Corrective Group | — | 17 | 1 | — | — | — |
| Chicago Control Group | 3 | 9 | — | — | — | — |
| Tampa Group | 1 | 11 | — | — | — | — |
| London Corrective Group | — | 14 | — | — | — | — |

The Mount Holyoke control group, the Tampa public speaking group and the London corrective group seem less subject to loss of voice for any cause than any of the other groups.   About one-third of the Mount Holyoke control group and one-twelfth of the Tampa group report in the affirmative.   Of the corrective groups, Mount Holyoke reports about one-sixth in the affirmative, Hunter corrective group one-half affirmative, while the San Francisco group reports about one-seventh affirmative. All of the Chicago corrective group reports in the negative, but a slightly affirmative trend is given for the control group as about one-fourth answer in the affirmative. Hysterical loss of voice has been reported by many writers, notably in England,[1] as being more frequent in girls than in men, whereas stuttering was found more frequently in men than in women.   It has even been suggested that perhaps aphonia or complete loss of voice is found, rather than stuttering, in women, and that it may represent much the same phenomenon.   There seems to be a somewhat greater tendency towards loss of voice in the woman's college corrective groups than in the control groups.   We find one-half or more of the Hunter College corrective group, but only one-fourth of the control group answering in the affirmative.

*Question 27.—Detecting off-key notes*

| Answers | Yes | No | Doubtful | Unans. |
|---|---|---|---|---|
| Mount Holyoke Corrective Group | 24 | 1 | — | — |
| Mount Holyoke Control Group   . | 227 | 29 | 2 | 1 |
| Hunter College Corrective Group | 24 | 1 | — | — |
| Hunter College Control Group   . | 24 | 1 | — | — |
| San Francisco Corrective Group . | 20 | — | 1 | 1 |
| Chicago Corrective Group .   . | 17 | 1 | — | — |
| Chicago Control Group   .   . | 12 | — | — | — |
| Tampa Group .   .   .   . | 11 | 1 | — | — |
| London Corrective Group .   . | 14 | — | — | — |

In all groups most of the answers are in the affirmative. In the largest, the Mount Holyoke control group, about

[1] Eileen MacLeod, King's College Hospital, London, 1931, *Lectures and Reports*, Speech Clinic (unpublished data).

one-tenth answer in the negative. The large number of positive answers is probably due to a better knowledge of music, more training, keener æsthetic judgment than was usual a generation ago. The results obtained from the Mount Holyoke and Hunter College corrective groups correspond closely to those found for all other groups, corrective or control.

*Question 28.—Noting differences in voices*

| Answers | Yes | No | Doubtful | Unans. | Total |
|---|---|---|---|---|---|
| Mount Holyoke Corrective Group | 18 | 7 | — | — | 25 |
| Mount Holyoke Control Group . | 227 | 28 | 1 | 3 | 259 |
| Hunter College Corrective Group | 23 | 2 | — | — | 25 |
| Hunter College Control Group | 24 | 1 | — | — | 25 |
| San Francisco Corrective Group | 21 | 1 | — | — | 22 |
| Chicago Corrective Group . | 17 | 1 | — | — | 18 |
| Chicago Control Group . . | 9 | 3 | — | — | 12 |
| Tampa Group . . . | 12 | — | — | — | 12 |
| London Corrective Group . | 14 | — | — | — | 14 |

The Mount Holyoke and the Chicago control groups as well as the Mount Holyoke corrective group are more conservative in answering the above question than are the others. The large number of answers in the affirmative in the Mount Holyoke, Chicago, San Francisco, and London corrective groups does not seem to correspond to the actual speech condition which we find in these groups. There seems to be some tendency to over-estimate the ability to note differences in speaking voices in these groups, as the actual possession of ability to discriminate between such variations ought normally to lead to individual correction of such difficulties by the student himself, and this seems not to have been the case. Perhaps the possession of a speech handicap renders the individual more critical of the voices around him, even though unable to eliminate his own speech defect. This might account for the larger number of positive answers given by all of the corrective groups. At any rate, the answer differs from what we should have expected in the corrective groups as contrasted with the non-speech defective or control groups.

### Question 29.—Noting differences in accent and pronunciation

| Answers | Yes | No | Unans. |
|---|---|---|---|
| Mount Holyoke Corrective Group . . | 24 | 1 | — |
| Mount Holyoke Control Group . . | 243 | 14 | 2 |
| Hunter College Corrective Group . . | 25 | — | — |
| Hunter College Control Group . . | 25 | — | — |
| San Francisco Corrective Group . . | 21 | — | 1 |
| Chicago Corrective Group . . . | 14 | 3 | 1 |
| Chicago Control Group . . . . | 12 | — | — |
| Tampa Public Speaking Group . . | 12 | — | — |
| London Corrective Group . . . | 14 | — | — |

The Mount Holyoke control and the Chicago corrective groups are the only ones which answer at all conservatively on the above questions. All of the other groups, corrective and control, express themselves as emphatically competent to detect differences in accent and pronunciation, most of the answers being in the affirmative.

### Question 30.—Dialectic ability and imitation

| Answers | Yes | No | Doubtful | Fair | Unans. |
|---|---|---|---|---|---|
| Mount Holyoke Corrective Group | 9 | 16 | — | — | — |
| Mount Holyoke Control Group . | 78 | 171 | 1 | 4 | 5 |
| Hunter College Corrective Group | 10 | 15 | — | — | — |
| Hunter College Control Group . | 11 | 14 | — | — | — |
| San Francisco Corrective Group . | 13 | 8 | 1 | — | 1 |
| Chicago Corrective Group . . | 8 | 10 | — | — | — |
| Chicago Control Group . . | 8 | 4 | — | — | — |
| Tampa Public Speaking Group . | 12 | — | — | — | — |
| London Corrective Group . . | 8 | 5 | — | — | — |

The largest number of answers in both the Mount Holyoke and Hunter College groups was in the negative in regard to ability to use dialect and to imitate voices. This was also true of the Chicago corrective group. The San Francisco and the London corrective groups as well as the Chicago control group, answer more frequently in the affirmative ; the Tampa public speaking group answers entirely in the affirmative. The latter being an organized public speaking class, its members are probably trained in the ability to imitate and to use dialect more effectively than are those in other groups, as the Mount Holyoke control group contains many students who have had no speech training. These replies would seem to indicate that the mere factor of training, even in speech correction, increases the student's ability along this line.

*Question* 31.—*Peculiarities in voice most readily noticed*

| Answers | Sound | Accent | Pronunciation | Foreign Accent; Dialect | Personality | Rate | Quality | Defects |
|---|---|---|---|---|---|---|---|---|
| Mount Holyoke Corrective Group . | 5 | 9 | 9 | 8 | 9 | — | — | — |
| Mount Holyoke Control Group . | 58 | 97 | 115 | 65 | 92 | — | — | — |
| Hunter College Corrective Group . | — | 14 | 5 | — | — | — | 20 | 3 |
| Hunter College Control Group . | — | 10 | 12 | 6 | — | — | 14 | — |
| San Francisco Corrective Group . | 8 | 9 | 9 | 6 | 9 | — | 1 | — |
| Chicago Corrective Group . . | — | 6 | 4 | 3 | 4 | — | 3 | — |
| Chicago Control Group . . | — | 2 | 5 | 2 | 2 | — | 1 | — |
| Tampa Public Speaking Group . | — | 3 | 3 | 1 | 7 | 2 | 6 | — |
| London Corrective Group . . | 4 | 4 | 4 | — | 2 | — | — | — |

Among other variations less frequently mentioned by the Mount Holyoke, Hunter College, and Tampa groups, were " tone " (tonal quality), lisping, harshness, nasality, stuttering, enunciation, shrillness, monotony, huskiness, and speech defects.

Less frequent variations noted by the public school groups in London corrective group were pitch, unpleasantness, harshness, coarseness, lisping and stuttering, assertiveness, firmness, affectation, and mispronunciation. A number of other descriptive terms were used, but not frequently enough to be considered as representative.

*Questions* 32 to 38 are concerned chiefly with discriminations made in regard to speech, voice and personality.

*Question 32.—Form of speech which seems to be easiest*

| Answers | Talking to Self | Talking in Group | To One Person | To Men | To Women | In Conversation | In Plays | Poetry | Prose | Argument |
|---|---|---|---|---|---|---|---|---|---|---|
| Mount Holyoke Corrective Group | 1 | 4 | 11 | 3 | 3 | 6 | 4 | 5 | 5 | 1 |
| Mount Holyoke Control Group | 11 | 40 | 89 | 9 | 20 | 78 | 37 | 57 | 64 | 7 |
| Hunter College Corrective Group | 5 | 6 | 6 | 1 | 1 | 12 | — | 4 | 6 | 2 |
| Hunter College Control Group . | 1 | 5 | 10 | 4 | 2 | 11 | 3 | 5 | 3 | 2 |
| San Francisco Corrective Group | 5 | 3 | 7 | 3 | 1 | 9 | 4 | 8 | 10 | 5 |
| Chicago Corrective Group . | 2 | 2 | 4 | 2 | — | 3 | 2 | — | 1 | 3 |
| Chicago Control Group . . | 1 | 1 | — | 2 | — | 7 | — | — | 1 | — |
| Tampa Public Speaking Group | — | 1 | 5 | 3 | 2 | 3 | — | 1 | 1 | 1 |
| London Corrective Group . | 6 | 2 | 2 | — | 1 | — | 1 | 3 | 3 | — |

As regards talking to self, to one person, or to a group, the highest frequencies of all were for the response "talking to one person", except in the Chicago control and the London corrective groups. In the Chicago control group no one answered the question regarding talking to one person, but one response each was given to indicate that it was easy to talk to a group or to oneself. The London corrective group marked "talking to oneself" most often. Most groups seem to find it easier to express oneself in conversation than to read poetry or prose, to take part in plays or in argument. The Mount Holyoke control group finds it easier to talk to women, and the Hunter College control group to men, but all of the public school groups and the Tampa group find it easier to talk to men. The London corrective group gives no responses under "talking to men" and only one response under "talking to women". The fact that the Mount Holyoke control and the Hunter College groups are in women's colleges, might explain the difference between the answers of these groups and of the public school and Tampa groups, but we find that an equal number of girls in the Mount Holyoke corrective group and in the same Hunter College group find it just as easy to talk to men as to women. The fact that the public schools represent a larger number of boys than girls, in these answers, is probably the chief reason why the answer " talking to men " is given with such frequency in the various groups. The Tampa group is about equally divided between the two, and in this group there are an equal number of men and women. Conversation, talking to one person, and speaking prose seem to be the favoured modes of communication.

*Question* 33.—*Do you judge people by the way they speak, dress or look ?*

In all except the Mount Holyoke control group the tendency is to judge people most frequently by the way they speak. The Mount Holyoke corrective group seems to judge more frequently by the way people " look ". The next highest frequency in all groups but the latter, is based on the " way people look ". Dress occupies the least important position in all of the judgments given.

*Question* 34.—*What are you able to tell about a person, by his voice or speech ?*

The answers listed by the Mount Holyoke control group of 259 members are arranged in order of frequencies :—

| | |
|---|---|
| Education | Moods |
| Culture or Refinement | Affectation |
| Personality | Forcefulness |
| Locality (from which the | Nervousness |
|     speaker comes) | Sense of Humour |
| Character | Interest in subject |
| Breeding | Reserve |
| Environment | Determination |
| Training | Emotionality |
| Intelligence | Sincerity |
| Interests | Politeness |
| Nationality | Type |
| Social status | Leadership |

In the Hunter College control group the highest frequencies in order were :—

Education
Environment and Culture
Personality
Character
Intelligence

Numerous other descriptive terms were given, but so infrequently that we have not attempted to classify them or to include them here.

The judgments listed by the corrective groups on this topic in order of frequency are :—

| Mount Holyoke | Hunter College | Mount Holyoke Under lesser frequencies we find |
|---|---|---|
| Education | Character | Intelligence |
| Personality | Environment | Background |
| Locality | Personality | Social adjustiveness |
| Culture | Culture | Effectiveness |
| Environment | Intelligence | Determination |
| Character | | Aggressiveness |
| Ease | | Dignity |
| Breeding | | Knowledge |
| Self-confidence | | |

A summary of the judgments of all other groups is practically impossible because of the wide divergence in type of answers, and they are therefore separately listed.

The San Francisco and London groups expressed themselves as able to tell the following things about the individual, by means of voice judgments :—

| San Francisco | London |
|---|---|
| Personality | Confidence |
| Culture | Intelligence |
| Richness of vocal quality | Determination |
| Depth of tones | Character |
| Determination | Clearness |
| Vigour | Humour |
| Intelligence | |

The Chicago corrective group placed their emphasis upon ability to judge of clearness, forcefulness, whether voice was kind, low-pitched, soft, pleasant, of good quality and plainly understood.

The Chicago control group stressed clearness, stimulating quality, drawling tones, pleasant quality, low pitch and intelligence shown.

The Tampa group stressed depth, power, ease and conviction in utterance, slow rate, softness of voice, personality, deliberation, character, smoothness, determination and interest.

Each of the above groups mentioned other character-

N

istics, but these were either duplications which have been included in the above, or terms which were analogous or infrequently given in the various reports.

Judgments such as personality, education and culture appear most frequently in these estimates, intelligence, vocal quality, terms referring to the mental attitude of the speaker and his manner of speaking, constituting most of the remaining responses.

*Question* 35.—Here the student was asked to mention the qualities of voice suggested to him by any particular speaker, or to recall some well-known voice with fairly well-marked characteristics, pleasant or otherwise, and to list such qualities as came to mind in judging that voice or speaker. Answers to this question overlapped with those found in the question just before it, and in giving the questionnaire again, it would be possible to combine these two questions to avoid duplication. One might then secure just as good an estimate of the student's judgment in regard to voice, personality and other characteristics of any speaker.

The answers to this question as given by the Holyoke and Hunter control groups are as follows, listed in order of frequency of occurrence :—

|  | Mount Holyoke Control Group |  | Hunter College Control Group |
|---|---|---|---|
| Culture | Kindness | Musical tones | Resonance |
| Clearness | Intelligence | Firmness | Personality |
| Forcefulness | Sympathy | Exactness | Clearness |
| Education | Depth | Energy and Vitality | Determination |
| Humour | Calmness | Resonance | Fluency |
| Determination | Will-power | Pronunciation | Self-confidence |
| Poise | Poise | Enunciation | |
| Personality | Sweetness [1] | Character | |
| Friendliness | Culture | Ambition | |

The answers given by the Mount Holyoke and Hunter College corrective groups, in order of frequency of occurrence, are as follows :—

[1] Such terms as " sweetness ", " kindness ", etc., are somewhat ambiguous, but these are the student's own expressions and convey meanings for which it is sometimes difficult to find a better word.

| Mount Holyoke Corrective Group | | Hunter College Corrective Group |
|---|---|---|
| Clearness | Monotony | Clearness |
| Culture | Well-organized material | Pleasing |
| Musical tones | Power in speech | Resonance |
| Personality | Kindness | Leadership |
| | Confidence | |

Clearness, culture, musical tones, personality and "kindness" are attributes which are common in the responses, in both of the Mount Holyoke lists.

For the public school and Tampa groups the characteristics listed may be summarized in order of frequencies as follows :—

| | |
|---|---|
| Softness | Education |
| Pleasant tones | Personality |
| Clearness | Self-control |
| Character (indications) | Quality |
| Culture | Kindness |
| Low pitch | Plain speech |
| Intelligibility | Pronunciation |

A number of other descriptive terms were used, but too seldom to be considered worthy of inclusion in this list. The wide range of variation in answers on the above questions is such that in giving such a questionnaire it is advisable to restrict the terms by suggesting a list of those such as appear most frequently in the above groups, and then to provide for a certain number of additional answers in case those suggested do not seem to apply.

The answers as given, however, are indicative of the speech and voice knowledge and interest on the part of students. They suggest some differences in discrimination, but this is probably because the Mount Holyoke control group is larger than the other groups, and is naturally expected to contain a wider variety of answers. The public school groups have stressed several characteristics which also appear in the Mount Holyoke and Hunter College lists, such as clearness, personality, pronunciation, culture, kindness, and vocal qualities. These are perhaps the qualities most frequently suggested to the listener when he attempts to make an estimate based upon the sound of the speaker's voice, or upon his personality and manner of speaking.

*Question 36.—Give several characteristics of the
pleasantest voice you know*

In the Mount Holyoke and Hunter College control groups
the characteristics were given in the following order :—

| Mount Holyoke | | Hunter College |
|---|---|---|
| Low-pitched | Mellow | |
| Clear | Animated | Well-modulated |
| Soft | Medium pitch | Good quality |
| Well-modulated | Flowing | Resonant—pitch variations |
| Good pitch variations | Vibrant | Clear—personality |
| Musical quality | Good quality | Determination |
| Smooth | Interesting | Fluency |
| Distinct | Rich | Self-reliance |
| Pleasing | Resonant | |
| Slow | Expressive | |
| Good enunciation | Quiet | |
| Good diction | | |
| Sweet | | |
| Moderate rate | | |

The high frequencies for the Mount Holyoke and
Hunter College corrective groups in order were :—

| Mount Holyoke | Hunter College |
|---|---|
| Soft | Resonant |
| Low | Well-modulated |
| Clear | Character and attitude |
| Musical | Environment |
| Distinct | Personality and culture |
| Well-modulated | Intelligence and fluency |
| Good pitch variations | Low-pitched |
| Enunciation | |
| Pronunciation | |

All of those terms listed most frequently in the corrective
group appear also in the control group above. A number
of varied terms appear, but so infrequently as to be
negligible for this summary.

The terms listed by all of the remaining groups, including
the San Francisco, Chicago corrective and control groups,
and Tampa group were as follows, in order of frequencies:—

| | | London Corrective Group |
|---|---|---|
| Soft | Pronunciation | Confidence |
| Clear | Richness | Intelligence |
| Pleasant | Depth | Character |
| Low-pitched | Evenness | Humour |
| Smooth | Slow rate | Distinctness |
| Good quality | Sweetness | Culture |
| | | Fluency |
| | | Good diction |

The characteristics listed in the first column above also appear in the first column for the Mount Holyoke control group, and several of them occur most frequently in the Mount Holyoke corrective group. There are no significant differences in other answers, except for the London corrective group, which includes a number of answers rarely mentioned in the responses of any of the other groups.

*Question 37.—Were you influenced by the voice, appearance, or personality of the person, in making your list of characteristics ?*

| Answers | Voice | Appearance | Personality | Total |
|---|---|---|---|---|
| Mount Holyoke Corrective Group | 11 | 1 | 12 | 24 |
| Mount Holyoke Control Group . | 113 | 9 | 115 | 237 |
| Hunter College Corrective Group | 12 | 1 | 12 | 25 |
| Hunter College Control Group . | 12 | 2 | 10 | 24 |
| San Francisco Corrective Group . | 12 | 4 | 6 | 22 |
| Chicago Corrective Group . . | 10 | 2 | 1 | 13 |
| Chicago Control Group . . | 3 | 2 | 3 | 8 |
| Tampa Public Speaking Group . | 5 | 1 | 5 (Unans. 1) | 12 |
| London Corrective Group . . | 6 | — | (Both, 4) 4 | 14 |

A number of students failed to answer the above question, apparently because of uncertainty as to the influence of these three factors upon their judgments. The Mount Holyoke and Hunter College corrective and control groups, the London corrective and the Tampa public speaking groups, were about equally divided in their answers between Voice and Personality. In the public school corrective groups the answers given most frequently were under the item *Voice*. The answers of the Chicago control group were almost evenly divided between voice, appearance and personality. In all groups the judgment has been influenced chiefly by voice and personality, and very little by the appearance of the speaker, evidently.

*Question 38.—What do you consider to be the chief characteristics of the cultured speech of the college man or woman ?* (Underline any of the following, or write additional answers, as) :—Well-modulated, smooth utterance, clearness in speech, intelligibility, good vocal quality, low pitch, moderate rate in speech, medium loudness, good variety in intonation, matter-of-fact tones, " plain " speech, decisive, crisp utterance, animated tones, etc.

CHIEF CHARACTERISTICS OF CULTURED SPEECH

| Answers | Well-modulated | Smooth | Clear | Intelligible or Plain | Good Vocal Quality | Low-pitched | Moderate Rate | Medium loud | Matter-of-fact Tones | Crisp or Decisive | Animated | Pitch Variations |
|---|---|---|---|---|---|---|---|---|---|---|---|---|
| Mount Holyoke Corrective Group . | 15 | 7 | 18 | 12 | 5 | 4 | 6 | 5 | — | 2 | 3 | |
| Mount Holyoke Control Group . . | 180 | 78 | 161 | 107 | 37 | 34 | 80 | 48 | 4 | 13 | 34 | 8 |
| Hunter College Corrective Group . | 25 | 16 | 19 | 14 | 11 | — | 10 | 5 | — | — | 3 | 1 |
| Hunter College Control Group . . | 20 | 9 | 18 | 12 | 10 | 4 | 7 | 7 | 3 | 3 | 4 | 1 |
| San Francisco Corrective Group . | 10 | 8 | 13 | 5 | 3 | 2 | 3 | 4 | 1 | 1 | 1 | |
| Chicago Corrective Group . . . | 4 | 3 | — | — | 1 | — | 1 | 1 | 1 | 1 | — | |
| Chicago Control Group . . . | 2 | — | 6 | 7 | — | — | 1 | — | — | — | 1 | — |
| Tampa Public Speaking Group . . | — | 4 | 4 | 5 | 1 | 1 | 2 | 3 | — | 1 | 1 | |
| London Corrective Group . . . | 2 | 2 | 4 | 1 | 5 | 1 | 1 | 1 | 2 | — | — | — |

In both the Mount Holyoke and the Hunter College groups the highest frequencies in responses were for well-modulated, clear, intelligible or plain speech and for pitch variations. This was also true of the San Francisco corrective group. In the Chicago corrective group *well-modulated* and *smooth* occupied first and second places, but in the Chicago control and the London corrective groups *intelligibility, clearness* and *vocal quality* occupied first and second places. In the Tampa group *intelligible, smooth, clear,* and *pitch variations* appeared most often. There is seen to be a high degree of similarity in the judgments on these points.    For the total number of responses given, we find the rank order to be as follows :—

| | |
|---|---|
| Well-modulated | Medium loud |
| Clear | Good vocal quality |
| Intelligible | Low-pitched |
| Pitch variations | Animated |
| Smooth | Crisp or decisive |
| Moderate rate | Matter-of-fact |

*Question 39.—Did you ever leave school because of your speech ?*

| Answers | Yes | No | Unans. | Totals |
|---|---|---|---|---|
| Mount Holyoke Corrective Group | 1 | 23 | 1 | 25 |
| Mount Holyoke Control Group  . | — | 257 | 2 | 259 |
| Hunter College Corrective Group | — | 24 | 1 | 25 |
| Hunter College Control Group  . | — | 25 | — | 25 |
| San Francisco Corrective Group . | — | 21 | 1 | 22 |
| Chicago Corrective Group  .    . | 2 | 16 | — | 18 |
| Chicago Control Group     .    . | — | 12 | — | 12 |
| Tampa Public Speaking Group  . | — | 12 | — | 12 |
| London Corrective Group  .    . | — | 14 | — | 14 |

Very few in any of the above groups have been compelled to leave school because of speech difficulty.    We find one who has done so, however, in the college corrective group and two in the Chicago corrective group.    A recheck on the unanswered questions indicates that none of those who failed to answer have had to leave school because of poor speech.    Out of the total number of responses given in all (348), only 3 students, or ·86, less than 1 per cent., have dropped out of school because of speech difficulty, and it is obvious that they have later re-entered.    These answers of course give us no indication as to the numbers who may have left school *permanently* because of speech difficulties.    Pupils with good intelligence, parental encouragement and sufficiently aggressive qualities may therefore tend to return to school, even though having left it once, because of speech difficulty, but from the lack of data as to the actual numbers who leave and who do not reappear in the school group, after leaving because of such difficulty, school records are inadequate and data scarce.    The very fact that in the above groups such students tend to remain in school and to make a struggle to remain there, is an additional argument for corrective measures and speech rehabilitation.

*Question 40.—Is your own speech good,*
*bad, or average ?* (fair)

| Answers | Good | Bad | Average or fair | Unans. | Total |
|---|---|---|---|---|---|
| Mount Holyoke Corrective Group | — | 3 | 21 | 1 | 25 |
| Mount Holyoke Control Group . | 25 | 2 | 226 | 6 | 259 |
| Hunter College Corrective Group | 1 | 5 | 19 | — | 25 |
| Hunter College Control Group . | 5 | 2 | 18 | — | 25 |
| San Francisco Corrective Group | 3 | 3 | 16 | — | 22 |
| Chicago Corrective Group . | 3 | 5 | 10 | — | 18 |
| Chicago Control Group . . | 4 | — | 8 | — | 12 |
| Tampa Public Speaking Group . | 1 | 1 | 10 | — | 12 |
| London Corrective Group . | — | 1 | 13 | — | 14 |

The highest frequencies in the Mount Holyoke control, Hunter College control, and Chicago control groups were (1) average, and (2) good. In the Mount Holyoke, Hunter College, Chicago, and London corrective groups, the highest frequencies were for (1) average, and (2) bad. In the San Francisco corrective and in the Tampa group the highest frequency was for *average*, while the responses for *good* and *bad* were equally divided. The speech-control groups seem to give a better subjective estimate of their own speech than do the corrective groups or the Tampa public speaking group. The statement therefore seems to be valid in such a questionnaire.

*Question 41.—Have you a pleasing voice ?*

This question is very similar to the one above, but was given to see which type of statement seemed to be best comprehended and most valid. It was less satisfactorily answered than the first, and it was necessary to arrange the answers under the headings :—

Yes    No    Fair    Doubtful    Unanswered

In all except the Tampa group the highest frequencies were for answers in the affirmative. The Tampa group was about equally divided between affirmative and negative. All groups except the Chicago control group had a scattering of answers under *fair, doubtful* or *un-answered*. The wording in Question 40 seems to be rather better for the purposes of self-rating, and to give the examiner a rough estimate of the student's own critical voice judgments so as to enable him at once to locate such students as possess noticeably bad voices, or who feel that their speech is particularly poor.

*Question 42.—Is your accent and pronunciation like that of most of your friends ?*

| Answers | Yes | No | Unans. |
|---|---|---|---|
| Mount Holyoke Corrective Group . . | 21 | 4 | — |
| Mount Holyoke Control Group . . | 222 | 27 | 10 |
| Hunter College Corrective Group . . | 19 | 5 | 1 |
| Hunter College Control Group . . | 22 | 3 | — |
| San Francisco Corrective Group . . | 14 | 6 | 2 |
| Chicago Corrective Group . . . | — | 17 | 1 |
| Chicago Control Group . . . | 7 | 4 | 1 |
| Tampa Public Speaking Group . . | 11 | 1 | — |
| London Corrective Group . . . | 9 | 5 | — |

In all groups there are at least some students who recognize differences between their own voices and those of their friends. While this question seems indefinite and probably too vague, it is interesting to note that in the Chicago corrective group all answers but one were " no ", indicating that all members are conscious of differences or variations between their own speech and the speech of their friends. Such answers therefore might have a bearing on the personality and social adjustment of the individuals concerned and be useful to the instructor in making an estimate of the student's speech and in planning corrective measures.

*Question 43.—If not, how does it differ ?*

In the Mount Holyoke and Hunter College corrective and control groups and in the Chicago corrective and control groups, the answer occurring most frequently was " accent ". In the San Francisco group the answers were about evenly divided between the responses *stuttering, pronunciation, cleft-palate speech, rapid speech,* and *tonal quality.* Tonal quality was the only adverse comment offered by the Tampa public speaking group regarding its speech, and responses were divided between *accent* and *tonal quality.*

" Accent " was the answer having highest frequency for all groups, with stuttering in second place. This indicates that foreign accent, local dialect, provincialism and pronunciation seem to be uppermost in the student's consciousness in answering this question, and to be the most frequent form of deviation in several of these groups ; stuttering comes second, and tonal quality or voice defects come third.

The remaining questions (44–48) are in regard to social adjustment and factors which might affect the personality of the individual, in relation to his speech development.

### Question 44.—*Are you a leader in your social group ?*

Total answers received, all groups :—

| Yes | No | Sometimes | Unanswered | Total Answers |
|-----|-----|-----------|------------|---------------|
| 211 | 167 | 13 | 22 | 413 |

In all except the Mount Holyoke control group, the largest number of answers was in the negative, showing lack of leadership qualities. The fact that the Mount Holyoke control group answered most frequently in the affirmative, gives this answer first place in the totals, but for all other groups the negative answer occurs most frequently. From the standpoint of personality it seems significant to the examiner that the corrective groups particularly stress this factor of lack of leadership in themselves.

### Question 45.—*Do you usually prefer to have someone else take the initiative in social activities ?*

This question is merely a different way of stating the same point as is mentioned in No. 44. The answers are so distributed between positive and negative in all but the Mount Holyoke control group, as to be indicative of very little. The answers were given under these headings :—

| Yes | No | Sometimes | Unanswered |
|-----|-----|-----------|------------|

A somewhat larger number in the Mount Holyoke and Hunter College control groups, and in the London corrective group answered " yes ", while in other groups the answers were very evenly divided between *yes* and *no*, with a scattering of *unanswered* and the response *sometimes*, so that this question seems less satisfactory than No. 44. In answering this question a number of the subjects expressed themselves as unwilling to be dominated, even though they were themselves unable to lead. It is possible that a negativistic attitude is even encouraged, by the fact of speech difficulty, so that the person finds it difficult to be co-operative or adjustive, even when help and encouragement are offered in corrective work.

*Question 46.—Have you ever felt inferior because of poor speech or personality ?*

| Yes | No | Sometimes | Unanswered | Total Answers |
|-----|-----|-----------|------------|---------------|
| 176 | 227 | 7 | 26 | 436 |

The majority of answers (227) were negative. The next highest were positive, with a few doubtful or unanswered. Answers from the groups which compare most favourably were from the Mount Holyoke, Hunter College, Chicago control groups, and the Tampa public speaking group. The majority of the answers in these cases were negative. The three corrective groups, Mount Holyoke, Chicago and San Francisco, gave a larger number of positive than negative answers. This seems to indicate that this question is useful and well worded, since it elicits the desired information, and the answers given correspond to known facts, as regarding the differences between corrective and control groups.

*Question 47.—Did you ever have any severe frights or shocks in childhood which in any way explain a possible speech difficulty, following same ?*

The total answers from all groups were as follows :—

| | Yes | No | Doubtful | Unans. |
|---|---|---|---|---|
| Mount Holyoke Corrective Group . | 2 | 22 | — | 1 |
| Mount Holyoke Control Group . | 2 | 247 | — | 10 |
| Hunter College Corrective Group | 2 | 23 | — | — |
| Hunter College Control Group . | 1 | 24 | — | — |
| San Francisco Corrective Group | 3 | 17 | 1 | 1 |
| Chicago Corrective Group . | 6 | 12 | — | — |
| Chicago Control Group . | — | 12 | — | — |
| Tampa Public Speaking Group . | — | 11 | — | 1 |
| London Corrective Group . | 3 | 11 | — | — |

In all except the Chicago control and the Tampa groups, there were a few answers in the affirmative, indicating that some shock or severe fright had been received which was of sufficient importance or vividness to be recalled very definitely in response to this question. One-third of the Chicago corrective group responded affirmatively to this question. While replies from the other groups were fewer, it is significant that such replies were received. They are explained to some extent in the answer to the last question.

*Question 48.—Explain the above in a brief statement*

| | Answers | No. of Cases |
|---|---|---|
| Mount Holyoke Control Group . | Wearing dental appliance which resulted in a lisp . . | 1 |
| | Terrified in unusual speech situation once . . . | 1 |
| | Embarrassing personal episode | 1 |
| Mount Holyoke Corrective Group | Shut in closet by mother as a punishment ; stutter began same day and has always persisted . . . . | 1 |
| | Embarrassing personal episode(?) (unsatisfactory explanation given, on rechecking) . . . . | 1 |
| Hunter College Control Group . | Intimidation in home in childhood associated with speech hesitation, which followed this incident . . | 1 |

| | Answers | No. of Cases |
|---|---|---|
| Hunter College Corrective Group | Severe illness, followed by neurotic lisp   .   .   . | 1 |
| | Fright causing hysterical loss of voice for several hours after punishment had been administered   .   .   . | 1 |
| San Francisco Corrective Group | Automobile accident   .   . | 1 |
| | Severe sting of a bee   .   . | 1 |
| | Shock from surgical operation | 1 |
| Chicago Control Group   .   . | None   .   .   .   .   . | — |
| Chicago Corrective Group   . | Fall from second-storey porch | 1 |
| | Fall and bruises in face .   . | 2 |
| | Frightened by snake   .   . | 1 |
| | Infantile Paralysis   .   . | 1 |
| Tampa Public Speaking Group . | None   .   .   .   .   . | — |
| London Corrective Group   . | Long illness and wasting sickness.   .   .   .   . | 1 |
| | Shock following surgical operation.   .   .   . | 1 |
| | Shaken by teacher for losing a paper, until arm was badly bruised, couldn't speak for several hours   .   .   . | 1 |

## Conclusions

The questionnaire has been found useful to the worker in speech correction and to the instructors in speech, as it enables the persons to whom the student is referred to look over the record which she made at the time of taking the speech tests, and the answers given on her questionnaire in regard to speech interests, special training, speech handicaps, and personality, are especially useful in advising or planning future work for the student. It also serves as a check upon the girl's attainment during her college course, and enables the instructor to find out to what extent she has improved her speech and general personality adjustments.

Some questions seem to more or less duplicate each other, and these may well be omitted in giving the questionnaire, as has been noted in the sections in which such questions have been analysed. The questionnaire does not duplicate the work of either the Personality Schedule, the personal data sheet for the Dean's office, or other data on file in the college offices, so that it serves a special purpose in connection with speech ability and interests, or special handicap in speech, and may be important in directing the student's development or enabling the instructor to better understand and to evaluate the student herself.

# CHAPTER IX

## PERSONALITY

### I. Thurstone Personality Schedule
### II. Trait Inventory

#### Personality Schedule

As a part of the work in speech correction the Thurstone Personality Schedule was given to two groups of Freshmen in the Fall of 1930 and in the Fall of 1931. It included all the students who were doing speech corrective work for the first semester of the years 1930 and 1931, or a total of 46 girls in the two groups.

As a control group for comparison, a class of 34 students, comprising all the students in Course 101, General Psychology, was used.[1] The result of the tests as given to the speech corrective groups does not differ widely from those given to the unselected group in Course 101, as may be seen by referring to the results. (Tables I and II.)

The scores obtained in the Scholastic Aptitude Tests were then correlated with the scores in Thurstone's Personality Schedule, and the latter was also correlated with scholarship. The results are given in Table III. The correlation between Personality Ratings and intelligence quotients compares favourably with that found by Thurstone, but he gives no general norms for Scholarship. The results obtained with our corrective groups, however, agree fairly well with those found for Mount Holyoke girls in Course 101, as shown in the table.

While the Thurstone Personality Schedule has been found to be better adapted to use in the corrective speech

[1] Steele, Isabel, " A Critical Study of Six Personality Tests," unpublished thesis submitted for Honours work, Mount Holyoke College, 1931, pp. 5–22.

groups than the Woodworth-Wells questionnaire or the Pressey X-O test, there is some difficulty in scoring, due to the fact that no provision is made for unanswered questions, which have therefore either to be all scored as negative, positive, or else omitted. The meaning of questions is not always clear, and there is no provision for any answer other than Yes or No.

Table V gives the answers arranged in order of highest frequencies, for those questions marked by 15 or more students from the two groups, and gives something of a composite picture of the two groups (p. 213).

| TABLE I | | | TABLE II | | |
|---|---|---|---|---|---|
| Range of Scores in Course 101 | | | Range of Scores for two Corrective Speech Groups, 1930 and 1931 | | |
| Score | | Per cent. of group | Score | | Per cent. of group |
| 13 | Emotionally well adjusted | 3 | 0 | | |
| — | | — | 6 | | |
| 19 | | | 8 | | |
| 21 | | | 12 | Emotionally well adjusted | 13 |
| 22 | | | 14 | | — |
| 23 | | | 14 | | |
| 26 | Well adjusted | 23 | — | | |
| 28 | | — | 16 | | |
| 28 | | | 17 | | |
| 29 | | | 18 | | |
| — | | | 19 | | |
| 31 | | | 21 | | |
| 34 | | | 22 | Well adjusted | 24 |
| 36 | | | 23 | | — |
| 37 | | | 24 | | |
| 38 | | | 24 | | |
| 38 | | | 26 | | |
| 41 | | | 29 | | |
| 45 | | | — | | |
| | (Median) 45–46 | | 30 | | |
| 46 | | | 30 | | |
| 46 | | | 31 | | |
| 48 | Average | 53 | 31 | | |
| 49 | | — | 32 | | |
| 50 | | | 32 | | |
| 51 | | | | (Median) 34 | |
| 59 | | | 36 | | |
| 59 | | | 38 | | |
| 59 | | | 39 | Average | 44 |
| 59 | | | 39 | | — |
| — | | | 39 | | |

<table>
<tr><td colspan="3">TABLE I—continued</td><td colspan="3">TABLE II—continued</td></tr>
<tr><td colspan="3">Range of Scores in Course 101</td><td colspan="3">Range of Scores for two Corrective<br>Speech Groups, 1930 and 1931</td></tr>
</table>

| Score | | Per cent. of group | Score | | Per cent. of group |
|---|---|---|---|---|---|
| 60 | | | 40 | | |
| 60 | | | 41 | | |
| 64 | Emotionally maladjusted | 18 | 42 | | |
| 70 | | — | 46 | | |
| 71 | | | 52 | | |
| 74 | | | 53 | | |
| — | | | 54 | | |
| 90 | Should have psychiatric advice | 3 | 56 | | |
| | | — | 57 | | |
| | | 100 | 59 | | |
| | | | — | | |
| | | | 61 | | |
| | | | 61 | | |
| | | | 64 | | |
| | | | 68 | | |
| | | | 70 | Emotionally maladjusted | 16 |
| | | | 74 | | — |
| | | | 78 | | |
| | | | — | | |
| | | | 83 | Needs psychiatric advice | 3 |
| | | | | | 100 |

Total number of students, 34
Range of scores, 13–90

Number of students, 46
Range of scores, 0–83

The Personality Scores as given by Thurstone [1] for diagnostic purposes are as follows :—

| Group | Personality Scores | Description |
|---|---|---|
| A | 0–14 | Extremely well adjusted |
| B | 15–29 | Well adjusted |
| C | 30–59 | Average |
| D | 60–79 | Emotionally maladjusted |
| E | 80– | Should have psychiatric advice |

While Thurstone found a reliability coefficient on the whole schedule which was very high (0·946), the correlation between the Personality Schedule and Intelligence was only 0·037, indicating that he found little in common between the scores in these two tests. In other words, we may expect to find superior or inferior intelligence as

[1] Thurstone, Personality Schedule, Univ. of Chicago Press, 1929 ed.

O

frequently among the neurotic as among the emotionally well-adjusted college students.[1]

The medians and range found for the Mount Holyoke corrective and control groups are compared with those found by Thurstone. (Table III.) [2]

### TABLE III

| | |
|---|---|
| Median for University of Chicago Freshmen on Thurstone Personality Schedule . . . . . . | 25–29 |
| Median for Mount Holyoke Control Group, Course 101 . . | 45–46 |
| Median for students in two speech Corrective Groups, 1930–1931 | 32–36 |
| Possible range of scores, Thurstone . . . . . | 0–223 |
| Range of scores for Chicago Freshmen . . . . | 5–134 |
| Range of scores for Mount Holyoke Control Group, Course 101 | 13–90 |
| Range of scores for Mount Holyoke Corrective Groups . . | 0–83 |

The scores in the Personality Schedules for the Mount Holyoke corrective groups and for the control group were correlated with the Scholastic Aptitude Test Scores and also with academic grades. These are given in Table IV.

### TABLE IV

#### CORRELATIONS [3]

| | I.Q. | Grades |
|---|---|---|
| Thurstone . . . . . | ·037 | — |
| Mount Holyoke (Course 101) . . | ·077 | ·24 |
| Mount Holyoke Corrective Groups . | ·006 | ·10 |

The results seem to justify the conclusion that the Personality Schedule does not touch upon the general factor of intelligence, but that both well-adjusted and poorly adjusted students may be found in the high-grade group in intelligence. The amount of positive correlation

---

[1] Thurstone, *Instructions for Using the Personality Schedule.*

NOTE.—Thurstone's test consists of 600 questions, to be used as a so-called " neurotic inventory ". The authors find that there seems to be " gradation between the psychopathological traits at one extreme through the neurotic indicators, to the more common forms of minor social and emotional maladjustments ".

Ref. Thurstone, " A Neurotic Inventory ", *Jour. of Soc. Psychol.*, Vol. I, 1, Feb. 1930, p. 13.

[2] Thurstone, L. and Th., *Instructions for Using Personality Schedule,* 1929, p. 3.

[3] Pearson's product-moment formula was used in computing the correlations.

found between grades and Personality Schedule is less than that quoted by others, who find more significant figures in the groups they have tested than we found in our two corrective groups, or in the control group. Pressey [1] has reported finding ·53 and ·33 while Guthrie [2] reports ·31 and ·51 from a similar study.

The slightly positive correlation for both Mount Holyoke groups, between scholarship (grades) and the Personality Schedule is in agreement with the findings of other investigators, and is mentioned by Thurstone, who compares personality scores and grades elsewhere. He accounts for his findings by assuming that neurotic students " are on the average better students than their well-adjusted classmates. The neurotic student has fewer social distractions than the well-adjusted student and he therefore concentrates more on scholastic attainment ". (Personality Schedule, Instr., p. 4.)

Thurstone finds that Freshman students, particularly, do not seem to falsify their answers, as judged by the intense seriousness with which they respond to the filling out of the questionnaire, and by later checks made as to adjustment. Even though some students answer more favourably than they seem to be warranted in doing, on the basis of apparent adjustment, their answers seem more reliable than any off-hand estimate of the individual's neurotic tendencies which might be obtained merely by studying facial expression, bearing, conversation or other overt forms of expression. The author feels that the sorting out of a number of students in need of psychiatric advice is a sufficient justification for the giving of the test.

The test as given to the speech corrective groups at Mount Holyoke in the Fall of 1930 and 1931 was not given for the purpose of finding those in need of psychiatric advice, primarily. It was given to aid the teacher in dealing with the student in individual speech conferences,

---

[1] Chambers, " Char. Traits and Prognosis of College Achievement ", *Jour. of Abnorm. Psychol. and Soc. Psy.*, 1925–26, Vol. 20, p. 308.

[2] Guthrie, E. R., " Measuring Introversion and Extroversion ", *Jour. Abnorm. Psy.*, 1927, Vol. 22, p. 84.

during some part of which it was possible to discuss any of the student's problems which might be in need of solution. While questions and a friendly attitude have not formerly been sufficient to draw out the student so as to enable the instructor to give the needed suggestions bearing on adjustment, it was found by means of the Personality Schedule that the students discussed quite freely the items which had been checked on the neurotic side of the scale. During both years we have found occasion to give the schedule at various times during the semester, depending somewhat upon the time element, progress in speech correction, or for other reasons. Each girl was given a conference varying from fifteen minutes to a full period, in going over her answers to the schedule. The readiness with which these students discussed the problems concerned, their frankness and obvious willingness to seek advice, was a surprise to the writer in nearly every case. One criticism on this procedure was that the conferences were delayed until near the end of the semester. The outcome of the interviews for both years convinced the writer that the schedule should be given early in the semester, and as near the beginning of the corrective work as possible, in order that constructive suggestions, analysis of the student's needs, therapeutic measures and mental catharsis may all be incorporated earlier in the work of speech correction, as an integral part of the training.

This would also enable the speech worker to get in touch with various other instructors who are in frequent contact with these students, to secure their co-operation. A certain amount of " mental hygiene " work may be applied by these instructors along with their regular conferences with these students. Not only is this possible with faculty members, but upper-classmen, " big sisters ", and various well-adjusted girls may be chosen to assist in improving the personality of certain girls, by taking special interest in them in the college halls, and by inviting them to participate in various college activities which the timid, self-conscious girl might otherwise shun.

Phillips,[1] in studying and treating the mental dangers of college students has found that unhappiness, due to internal conflicts for which the student himself has found no solution, often come to the surface in interviews with sympathetic, understanding teachers or with older students. He finds that unfortunately such conflicts are dismissed sometimes by faculty and students " with a gesture and a smile ".  He calls such an attitude on the part of faculty or older students a psychological problem in itself, indicating a wrong, biased, or non-sympathetic point of view.

The schedule consists of 223 questions, and the maximum score would be 223, provided every question were answered unfavourably.  There are questions relating to the subject's family life, sex life, position in family, or order of birth.  Lack of rapport between imagination and reality are included, since the authors believe that " the fundamental characteristic of the neurotic personality is an imagination that fails to express itself effectively on external social reality ".*

The following table gives the list of questions which were answered unfavourably by the largest number of students.  At the left they are numbered in rank order, and at the right are given the frequencies for each of these answers.  It does not include all of the questions given in the questionnaire, but only such as have been answered by the largest numbers of students, ranging from 13–29 answers.

TABLE V

THURSTONE PERSONALITY SCHEDULE

| Rank Order | | Frequencies |
|---|---|---|
| 1 | *Do you find it difficult to speak in public ? . . | Yes—29 |
| 2 | *Do you often feel self-conscious in the presence of superiors ? . . . . . . . | Yes—28 |
| 3 | *Do you day-dream frequently ? . . . . | Yes—26 |
| 5 | Do you say things on the spur of the moment and then regret them ? . . . . . . | Yes—23 |
| | *Do you get stage fright ? . . . . . | Yes—23 |
| | *Do you hesitate to volunteer in a class recitation ? . | Yes—23 |

---

[1] Phillips, D. E., " Mental Dangers Among College Students ", *Jour. of Abnormal Psychology*, Vol. 25, 1, Apr.-June 1930, p. 3.

* Items with star appear in Thurstone's " Neurotic Inventory ", *ibid.*, p. 27.

Thurstone Personality Schedule—*continued*

Rank
Order                                            Frequencies

7
- *Do you have difficulty in starting conversation with a stranger?  .  .  .  .  .  .  .  Yes—22
- Do you allow people to crowd ahead in line?  .  .  Yes—21
- *Do you get discouraged easily?  .  .  .  .  Yes—21

10
- *Does it bother you to have people watch you at work even when you do it well?  .  .  .  .  Yes—21
- *Do you have ups and downs in mood without apparent cause?  .  .  .  .  .  .  .  .  Yes—21
- Are you sometimes the leader at a social affair?  .  No—21
- *Have you ever been depressed because of low marks in school?  .  .  .  .  .  .  .  Yes—20

14
- *Do you lack self-confidence?  .  .  .  .  .  Yes—20
- Are you regarded as indifferent to the opposite sex?  Yes—20

18
- *Do you often feel lonesome, even when you are with other people?  .  .  .  .  .  .  Yes—19
- At a reception or tea do you seek to meet the important person present?  .  .  .  .  .  No—19
- Are you slow in making decisions?  .  .  .  .  Yes—19
- Can you stand disgusting smells?  .  .  .  .  No—19
- *Do your feelings alternate between happiness and sadness without apparent reason?  .  .  .  .  Yes—19

23
- Are your day-dreams about improbable occurrences?  Yes—18
- *Are your feelings easily hurt?  .  .  .  .  Yes—18
- *Are you troubled with feelings of inferiority?  .  Yes—18
- *Are you in general self-confident about your abilities?  No—18
- *Are you troubled with shyness?  .  .  .  .  Yes—18

27·5
- *Do you worry too long about humiliating experiences?  Yes—17
- Do you like to be by yourself a great deal?  .  .  Yes—17
- Do you ever have a queer feeling as if you were not your old self?  .  .  .  .  .  .  Yes—17
- Are you afraid of falling when you are on a high place?  Yes—17

30·5
- *Are you easily moved to tears?  .  .  .  .  Yes—16
- *Do you often experience periods of loneliness?  .  Yes—16

33
- If you came late to a meeting, would you rather stand or leave than take a front seat?  .  .  .  Yes—15
- *Do you consider yourself a rather nervous person?  .  Yes—15
- Do you ever take the lead to enliven a dull party?  .  No—15

35·5
- *Do you often feel just miserable?  .  .  .  .  Yes—14
- As a child did you like to play alone?  .  .  .  Yes—14

39·5
- Have you found books more interesting than people?  Yes—13
- Are you ever bothered by a feeling that things are not real?  .  .  .  .  .  .  .  .  Yes—13
- Do you make friends easily?  .  .  .  .  .  No—13
- *Do you ever have spells of dizziness?  .  .  .  Yes—13
- *Do you keep in the background on social occasions?  .  Yes—13
- *Do ideas often run through your head so that you cannot sleep?  .  .  .  .  .  .  Yes—13

---

* Items with star appear in Thurstone's "Neurotic Inventory", *ibid.*, p. 27.

The questions contain items regarding the subject's family, such as " Were your parents happily married ? " ; questions concerning the subject's sex life and socialization such as " Do you limit your friendships mostly to your own sex ? " ; questions as to position in the family, such as " Were you your parents' favourite child ? " The questions which are starred in our list of high-frequency answers are those which are designated by Thurstone as the most differentiating questions in the Personality Schedule. Sixty per cent. of the significant questions listed by Thurstone appear above in our list of high-frequency answers. This in itself is a strong argument for the need of mental hygiene as well as corrective speech work with these students.

## REFERENCES

Allport and Vernon, *A Study of Values.* (Scale for Measuring Dominant Interests.)

Allport, G. W., and F. H., *A–S Reaction Study.*

Downey, *Will-Temperament Test.*

Freyd, M., " Introverts and Extroverts ", *Psychological Review*, 1924, Vol. 31.

Laird, D. Colgate, " Tests of Emotional Outlets ", *Personal Inventory*, C 2 ; *ibid.*, C 3 ; *ibid.*, B 2.

Mental Survey Scales, Indiana Univ. Dept. of Psychology, *Schedule E, Test IV, Moral Judgment.*

Pressey-Pressey, S. and L., *X–O Tests*, Test 4, p. 4.

Woodworth-Wells, *Questionnaire*, Columbia University, N.Y.

Stinchfield, *Speech Questionnaire for Adults and College Students*, No. 17098, Speech tests.

## TRAIT INVENTORY

In addition to the Thurstone Personality Schedule a Trait Inventory was arranged by the writer and given to three groups of Freshmen in the Fall of 1926. This consisted of a list of forty-six desirable and undesirable traits, or those which might be classed as favourable or unfavourable according to their relationship to other personality traits, and which altogether might give the worker a better understanding of the individual than could be obtained from the Personality Schedule alone, or from personal conferences only. It was felt that it would be necessary to analyse the results for a special group and for a control group, in order to ascertain whether the trait list yielded any important results, and to determine which traits, if any, were of greatest importance in the list.

The trait list was given to all Freshman girls in the Fall of 1926, and has since been given frequently to other corrective groups, because of the findings on the initial use of the list. The three groups to whom the list was given consisted of 33 subjects from the class, who had been classified for speech corrective work, 33 subjects from the same class, who had superior speech, and to all of the remaining members of the class, consisting of 204 subjects who were neither corrective subjects nor in the superior speech group, and who therefore consisted of those of " average " attainment in speech.

The forty-six traits are arranged in rank order for the corrective group, according to the frequency with which answers in the affirmative occurred. The results for Groups II and III (Control and Average Groups) are placed in the corresponding column for purposes of comparison. The list of traits is not all-inclusive, but is a selective one, arranged to assist the speech teacher in understanding the personality of these students, and to facilitate practical corrective measures in speech and personality.

### TRAIT INVENTORY

A list of 46 traits given to three groups in the Fall of 1926.
Group   I. Corrective Speech Groups, 33 subjects.
Group  II. Superior Speech Group, 33 subjects (control group).
Group III. Average Speech Group, consisting of the remaining 204 subjects in this freshman class.
The trait list is arranged in order of frequency of responses which were given by Group I. The percentages given by the other groups are placed opposite for purposes of comparison.

| Trait to be underlined by Student | Percentage of Responses in | | |
|---|---|---|---|
| Rank Order (Group I) | Group I | Group II | Group III |
| 1 Co-operative   .   .   . | 88 | 94 | 92 |
| 2 Eager   .   .   .   . | 70 | 73 | 83 |
| Independent   .   .   . | 70 | 67 | 70 |
| Cheerful   .   .   .   . | 70 | 76 | 75 |
| 4·5 Democratic   .   .   . | 70 | 91 | 88 |
| Optimistic .   .   .   . | 70 | 82 | 77 |
| Imitative   .   .   .   . | 70 | 12 | 39 |

## TRAIT INVENTORY—*continued*

| Trait to be underlined by Student | Percentage of Responses in | | |
|---|---|---|---|
| Rank Order (Group I) | Group I | Group II | Group III |
| 8 Practical . . . . | 61 | 82 | 76 |
| Even disposition . . . | 52 | 73 | 67 |
| Courteous . . . . | 52 | 94 | 88 |
| Quiet . . . . | 52 | 73 | 70 |
| 12 Good memory . . . | 52 | 55 | 59 |
| Well-controlled . . . | 52 | 79 | 67 |
| Not over-sensitive . . | 52 | 58 | 67 |
| Subject to day-dreaming . | 52 | 20 | 63 |
| Aggressive . . . . | 33 | 27 | 28 |
| Tactful . . . . | 33 | 70 | 56 |
| Self-centred . . . | 33 | 34 | 27 |
| Make contacts easily . . | 33 | 70 | 67 |
| Close-mouthed . . . | 33 | 36 | 38 |
| 21·5 Easily satisfied . . . | 33 | 67 | 68 |
| Calm . . . . | 33 | 61 | 48 |
| Tactless . . . . | 33 | 18 | 28 |
| Communicative . . . | 33 | 49 | 47 |
| Unselfish . . . . | 33 | 46 | 58 |
| 26 Original . . . . | 30 | 46 | 39 |
| Prosaic . . . . | 18 | 27 | 19 |
| Moody . . . . | 18 | 18 | 21 |
| Forgetful . . . . | 18 | 36 | 33 |
| Afraid to meet people . . | 18 | 21 | 22 |
| 31·5 Very emotional . . . | 18 | 9 | 17 |
| Often dissatisfied . . | 18 | 24 | 20 |
| Very sensitive . . . | 18 | 24 | 25 |
| Snobbish . . . . | 18 | 6 | 4 |
| Often worried . . . | 18 | 30 | 38 |
| Cynical . . . . | 18 | 9 | 10 |
| 37 Retiring . . . . | 17 | 15 | 55 |
| 38 Quick tempered . . . | 12 | 24 | 25 |
| Selfish . . . . | 9 | 27 | 24 |
| 40·5 Dependent . . . . | 9 | 18 | 18 |
| Poor manners . . . | 9 | 3 | 2 |
| Noisy . . . . | 9 | 21 | 18 |
| Indifferent . . . . | —* | 9 | 8 |
| 44·5 Impractical. . . . | —* | 15 | 11 |
| Impersonal . . . | —* | 39 | 43 |
| Unco-operative . . . | —* | —* | 1·9 (1·9 per cent.) |

\* Unanswered.

## *Variations in Responses of the Three Groups*

While we are somewhat sceptical about the scoring of personality traits by the students themselves, in a list of this type, we were surprised to find that the corrective group had checked off a considerable number of questionable or negative traits, as compared with the superior speech group and the average group.

It may be that it is not important to give any such rating to average or superior students, but so many of the girls in the corrective group actually scored themselves unfavourably or on questionable traits, with a high degree of honesty, as later records and studies actually indicated, that we feel that such a trait list is of considerable use and importance in making a preliminary study of the personality of girls in a corrective group. We have therefore used this list rather frequently from time to time, for this purpose.

The corrective group responses indicate that these students feel that they tend to be less co-operative than are better adjusted girls. This fact is important in life relationships. The girls in Groups II and III rate themselves as more cheerful than the girls in Group I ; also as more democratic and more optimistic. A considerably smaller number of girls in the corrective group marked themselves " practical " than in the other two groups.

In all of the following traits the girls in the corrective group rated themselves below both of the other groups, by a considerable margin in most instances :—

> Even disposition
> Courteous
> Quiet
> Good memory
> Well-controlled (emotionally)
> Not over-sensitive

In both the corrective and the average group there seem to be many more " day-dreamers " than in the best-adjusted speech group, there being only 20 per cent. of responses in the superior speech group.

The girls in the corrective group have rated themselves as somewhat more aggressive than the other two groups, but the difference is slight. This may indicate some attempt at over-compensation for a real or fancied personality shortcoming.

A surprisingly small number of girls in the corrective group rated themselves as " tactful ". Almost twice as many girls scored themselves favourably on this point in the other two groups. This is significant in social communication, and is a personality trait which the Group I girls could well afford to develop. A smaller number of girls in the average group have rated themselves self-centred than in either the corrective or the control group, but the difference is not a large one and is perhaps unimportant. Under the heading " tactless ", the smallest number of responses is given by the well-adjusted or superior speech group, the next largest by the average group, and the largest number of responses by the girls in the corrective group. This corresponds roughly with the rating they have already given themselves regarding " tact ", above.

It is significant that in each of the following traits the girls in the corrective group rate themselves lowest, viz. :—" Do you make contacts easily ; are you close-mouthed, easily satisfied, calm, communicative, unselfish, original ? " The superior speech group takes highest rating on trait " prosaic ". This agrees with the higher rating which they give themselves under the heading " practical ", also. In moodiness or tendencies towards the same the groups correspond closely, as rated. The corrective group does not claim to be specially " forgetful ", while about one-third of those in the other two groups do so rate themselves. We may question this rating, because according to psychology, the very presence of a speech defect, often tends to make the student less talkative and more subject to lapses of memory than when no such difficulty exists.

The speech corrective group does not differ widely from the other two groups in willingness to meet people. Fear of social contacts and of meeting people is probably more typical of the stutterer than of other people possessing a speech handicap, but even then the desire to meet people easily and normally is present in a high degree in the stutterer, even in the face of apparent contradictions in his personality, we find.

Both the corrective and the average groups mark themselves as more emotional than do the girls in the superior speech group. Emotional control and poise seem to be possessed in the highest degree in the superior speech group. The tendency to feel dissatisfied and to be sensitive seems to be found to a higher degree in the average and superior speech groups, according to their own evaluation. Tendency to worry is found also in these two groups more than in the corrective group. The greater passivity of the girls possessing a speech defect, and tendency to take the background socially, may account for this difference in answers. It seems significant that the corrective group marks itself as more snobbish and more cynical than do either of the other two groups.

The stimulus word for " retiring " or " reticence " is apparently a poor one, since the girls in the average group rate themselves highest on this trait, the other two groups grading themselves about equally. We feel that this word may be poorly chosen, unless it is possible that the possession of a speech handicap, and the possession of superior speech, both tend to stimulate the individual to make greater social efforts, and that the girl in the corrective group may over-compensate for a fancied inferiority by being or seeming more aggressive than she really is, in order to conceal a personality flaw which might be unfavourable. The girls in the corrective group rate themselves lower than either of the other two groups on the traits quick-temper, selfishness, dependency, tendency to be noisy. The corrective group rates lowest on *manners*, giving themselves more of a penalty than do either of the other groups.

The corrective group did not rate itself on the following items:—indifference, impracticality, impersonality and lack of co-operation. The other two groups rated themselves on all of these items with the exception of "unco-operative", on which the superior group failed to make any record.

While some of these traits more or less duplicate each other, both are helpful in giving us a fair estimate of the personality of the student, and as the traits are not placed opposite each other, so that the favourable and unfavourable, or desirable and undesirable ones may be too easily identified as such, one is able to secure fairly good cooperation from the markers, we feel, inasmuch as some important and apparently significant differences appear in the self-ratings of these three groups, which may be applied by the teacher as a part of her training in speech and personality, in dealing with students in the speech-correction group.

# CHAPTER X

## HANDEDNESS

RECENT clinical studies in handedness, particularly those by Orton,[1] Travis,[2] and Jasper,[3] are in support of the Cerebral Dominance theory, according to which they have found that in many cases of stuttering there is a reduction in cortical lead-control which results in a neuro-muscular derangement. This derangement is manifest in blocking, hesitancy, or stuttering. Lack of dominance by one hemisphere, or one centre, leads to transient inhibitive tendencies, so that the stutterer is employing both hemispheres of relatively equal potential energy, in the motor control called for in speech. Rivalry between the two hemispheres may result in speech which ranges from complete blocking, to stuttering or mild hesitation, according to this theory.

In order to compare the various researches in this field with indications of dextrality and sinistrality in the speech corrective group at Mount Holyoke, the basis of selection for indices of handedness used was Jasper's inventory,[4] which is a part of the battery of clinical tests in use in the Iowa Speech Clinic.

Twenty-five Freshmen held for speech correction in the Fall of 1931 were given the inventory, and were then compared with a control group consisting of twenty-five girls from a superior speech group, representing students

[1] Orton, S. T., " Studies in Stuttering ", IV, *Arch. Neurol. and Psychiat.*, 21, 1929, pp. 61–8.
  Travis, L. E., " Studies of Action Currents in Stutterers ", *Arch. Neurol. and Psychiat.*, 21, 1929, pp. 61–8.
[2] Travis, L. E., *Speech Pathology*, 1931, pp. 95–192.
[3] Jasper, H. H., " Neuro-Muscular Organization in Stutterers ", Iowa Univ. Studies in Psychology, XV, Psycholog. Monog., Vol. XLIII, 1, 1932, pp. 72–174.
[4] Jasper, *ibid.*, pp. 172–4.

in elective courses, who had had more than one course in speech. The number of stutterers held for speech correction in Mount Holyoke College in any single year is so small that it was felt the study should include also a group of speech correctives and a group of girls of superior speech.

The reason for this choice was the writer's feeling that in cases where actual stuttering is not present, but where there is confusion in thought, slow, deliberate speech, poor motor control, lisping, slovenly speech, it seems possible that a lack of cerebral dominance in such cases might be indicated by the findings of such an index, even though all students included in such a study might not be actual stutterers.

The inventories were given and results tabulated with the assistance of Miss Lucile McLaughlin, Psychology Major during the year 1931–32. The results are set forth in Tables I, II, III, and IV.

## Procedure

The handedness inventories were given out to all members of the corrective group at the time of a required conference, and each girl was asked to take home the inventory, and to check up by self-observation during the week, on points which she found herself unable to answer without such observation. Similar instructions were given to the group representing the superior or control group. Replies were tabulated for twenty-five Freshmen corrective group members, and for the twenty-five whose questionnaires were first returned from the superior group, making a total of fifty studies used.

Following the custom used by the originator of the questionnaire, the score was found by subtracting the percentage of all items answered " left " from the percentage of all items answered " right ". A " positive " score represents a majority of right-hand preferences, a zero score indicates an equal proportion of right- and left-hand preferences, or ambidexterity. A negative score indicates a majority of left-hand preferences.

In the unselected group studied by Jasper about 6 per cent. fell below zero, this being about the percentage of sinistrality usually found in an unselected group. Our classification was as follows :—

| No. of Students | | |
|---|---|---|
| 25 | Right-handed normals . . | RN |
| 25 | Speech correction group . | CORR |
| 4 | Stutterers . . . . | S |

In our two groups the entire fifty subjects claimed to be right-handed, but two were right-handed-changed, and if classified according to Jasper's method of selection of subjects, these two would have been placed in his LN group. Granting that these subjects were native-left-handed individuals, it would give a total of 4 per cent. of left-handed subjects in the total number studied, which is not far below the amount found by Jasper in his larger experimental group.

The two possibly left-handed individuals in our groups were not stutterers. Neither one was a well-adjusted personality, and the scholarship was low in both cases. This seems to point to the inference that handedness, even though not initiating a speech defect, may be linked with general maladjustment, poor motor co-ordination and disharmony. Out of the entire number of correctives, controls and stutterers, we found only two instances of LN subjects. One of these was in the normal speech group, and one in the group of speech correctives, but neither case was found in the group of stutterers.

TABLE I

Showing comparison between total speech corrective group and superior speech group on handedness index. Total, 50 subjects

RN—Right-handed normal, superior speech group
CORR—Speech correction group
R—Right-handed
L—Left-handed
X—Ambidextrous

| | | R Per cent. | L Per cent. | X Per cent. |
|---|---|---|---|---|
| RN | . | 75 | 7·3 | 17·7 |
| CORR | . | 76·62 | 7·80 | 15·56 |

This table indicates that there is very little difference between the findings for the Corrective and for the Superior Speech group on the basis of handedness in all of the activities listed. There is a slightly higher percentage of ambidexterity indicated in the superior speech group. The percentages of right- and left-handedness do not show so wide a variation as might have been anticipated, the corrective group even rating slightly higher than the RN group on right and left dominance. It must be borne in mind that the Corrective group does not consist of stutterers only.

TABLE II

Showing a comparison between the control (superior speech) group and stutterers in class examined in Fall of 1931

RN—Control group (25 subjects) superior speech
S—Stutterers [1] (4 subjects) corrective speech

|  | R<br>Per<br>cent. | L<br>Per<br>cent. | X<br>Per<br>cent. |
|---|---|---|---|
| RN . . | 75 | 7·3 | 17·7 |
| S . . | 78·5 | 9 | 12·5 |

In the above group we find a higher percentage of right-handed stutterers and of normal speech subjects than were found by Travis and Jasper (p. 77). There is a higher percentage of left-handedness in the stutterers' group than in the superior speech group, however. The percentage of ambidexterity is higher in the superior speech group than in the corrective group, and does not match the findings in regard to left-handedness for the two groups. It is significant that the findings definitely indicate a greater amount of left-handedness in the speech corrective group, even though the number of stutterers in the class were so few that one might have expected the results to be negative, on this point.

While our findings agree with those of Travis and his colleagues in regard to greater amount of left-handedness in stutterers as compared with a superior speech group or

[1] Four stutterers represented the entire number having this type of speech difficulty in the class examined in the Fall of 1931, the remaining girls in the corrective group being held for causes other than stuttering.

P

with a corrective group, we find fewer indications of ambidexterity than they have shown, and the percentage of left-handedness is less, as a whole.

Cerebral dominance, therefore, as applied to stuttering seems to have important implications on the basis of handedness as shown in Table II, but as applied to speech defects other than stuttering, the index cannot be said to be significant, since interference with cerebral dominance seems not to be related to such speech defects as lisping, oral inaccuracy and letter-substitution.

A further study of these subjects was made as to eye and ear preferences and muscle dominance in certain activities. These are given in the following tables.

### TABLE III

1. EYE PREFERENCE.

Eye generally used in sighting, gauging distance, aiming gun, etc.

Key { RN—Superior speech group (25 subjects)
CORR—Speech correction group (25 subjects)
S—Stutterers (4 subjects)

| | R No. | R Per cent. | L No. | L Per cent. | X No. | X Per cent. | Total Per cent. |
|---|---|---|---|---|---|---|---|
| RN | 15 | 83·5 | 2 | 11 | 1 | 5·5 | 100 |
| CORR | 12 | 67 | 6 | 33 | 0 | — | 100 |
| S | 2 | 50 | 2 | 50 | 0 | — | 100 |

It is interesting to note that eye dominance of the superior speech group is stronger in the right eye, whereas both the corrective and the stutterer groups show a greater amount of left-eye dominance than does the superior speech group. Half of the responses in the stutterers' group are for left-eye dominance.

2. EAR DOMINANCE.

Ear usually turned in the direction of sounds.

| | R No. | R Per cent. | L No. | L Per cent. | X No. | X Per cent. | Total Per cent. |
|---|---|---|---|---|---|---|---|
| RN | 10 | 40 | 5 | 20 | 10 | 40 | 100 |
| CORR | 7 | 28 | 2 | 8 | 16 | 64 | 100 |
| S | 1 | 25 | 1 | 25 | 2 | 50 | 100 |

In the superior speech group (RN) there is an equal number of responses for right-ear dominance and dominance by either ear. In the corrective and stutterers' groups, however, there is a higher percentage of responses under ambidexterity than for right- or left-ear dominance. There is an equal number of responses for right- and left-ear dominance in the stutterers' group.

3. MUSCLE DOMINANCE and handedness in such activities as throwing ball, swinging bat, shuffling cards, turning pages of book, using tennis racquet.

A. *Throwing Ball.*

| | R | | L | | X | | Total |
|---|---|---|---|---|---|---|---|
| | No. | Per cent. | No. | Per cent. | No. | Per cent. | Per cent. |
| RN | 25 | 100 | 0 | — | 0 | — | 100 |
| CORR | 24 | 100 | 0 | — | 0 | — | 100 |
| S | 4 | 100 | 0 | — | 0 | — | 100 |

All groups definitely right-handed in this performance.

B. *Swinging Bat.*

| | R | | L | | X | | Total |
|---|---|---|---|---|---|---|---|
| | No. | Per cent. | No. | Per cent. | No. | Per cent. | Per cent. |
| RN | 23 | 92 | 1 | 4 | 1 | 4 | 100 |
| CORR | 24 | 100 | 0 | — | 0 | 0 | 100 |
| S | 3 | 75 | 0 | — | 1 | 25 | 100 |

C. *Shuffling Cards.*

| | R | | L | | X | | Total |
|---|---|---|---|---|---|---|---|
| | No. | Per cent. | No. | Per cent. | No. | Per cent. | Per cent. |
| RN | 18 | 72 | 0 | 0 | 7 | 28 | 100 |
| CORR | 18 | 75 | 6 | 25 | 0 | 0 | 100 |
| S | 2 | 50 | 0 | 0 | 2 | 50 | 100 |

In swinging the bat 92 to 100 per cent. use the right hand in both the superior speech group and in the corrective group. Among the stutterers only 75 per cent. (three out of four) use the right hand, the remaining 25 per cent. being ambidextrous.

D. *Turning Pages.*

| | R | | L | | X | | Total |
|---|---|---|---|---|---|---|---|
| | No. | Per cent. | No. | Per cent. | No. | Per cent. | Per cent. |
| RN | 17 | 68 | 1 | 4 | 7 | 28 | 100 |
| CORR | 21 | 84 | 4 | 16 | 0 | 0 | 100 |
| S | 3 | 75 | 1 | 25 | 0 | 0 | 100 |

In turning the pages of a book we find that 28 per cent. of the superior speech group use either hand, 4 per cent. are left-handed and 68 per cent. right-handed in the performance. In the corrective group we find 16 per cent. are left-handed, none ambidextrous, but 84 per cent. use the right hand in this activity. In the stutterers' group we find one out of four to be left-handed in this activity (25 per cent. of the total), and three are definitely right-handed (75 per cent.) in turning pages. While we find no ambidexterity in the corrective group and the group of stutterers, we do find a higher percentage of left-handedness than in the superior speech group.

E. *Swinging Tennis Racquet.*

|  | R | | L | | X | | Total |
|---|---|---|---|---|---|---|---|
|  | No. | Per cent. | No. | Per cent. | No. | Per cent. | Per cent. |
| RN | 25 | 100 | 0 | 0 | 0 | 0 | 100 |
| CORR | 24 | 100 | 0 | 0 | 0 | 0 | 100 |
| S | 4 | 100 | 0 | 0 | 0 | 0 | 100 |

The question in regard to use of the tennis racquet gives negative results, as 100 per cent. of all subjects use the right hand in playing tennis.

In order to compare our results with Travis' norms for left-handed normal individuals (without speech defects) it would be necessary to have a fairly large and well-equated group, but we found only one left-handed-changed individual in each of the two groups, viz. : superior speech group and corrective speech group, so far as student's own testimony and the results of the inventory were reliable. For these two subjects the findings were as follows :—

Superior speech group I LN score 19 ; right-handed-changed. Poor scholarship ; not a stutterer ; poorly adjusted ; in elective speech course.

Corrective speech group I LN score 44 ; right-handed-changed. Not a stutterer ; poor social adjustment ; poor scholarship.

Range of scores in superior speech group of 25 subjects, 19–66. Excluding the one case of left-handedness, the scores run 26–66 in this group.

Range of scores in the corrective speech group of 25 subjects, 29–66. The one case of right-handed-changed had a score of 44 as already reported, and was not a stutterer.

Range of scores for the 4 stutterers in this year's class, 29–60. No right-handed-changed individuals found.

The scores were obtained by subtracting the percentage of all left items from percentage of all items answered " right ". Zero score would mean an equal number of " right " and " left " answers. A negative score would mean a majority of left-handed preferences were shown. We found no negative or zero scores in either of our two equated groups, viz. : the superior speech and the corrective group consisting of a total of 50 subjects. The scores were all positive, that is, showed more right-hand preferences than left-hand or ambidextrous tendencies.

This brings up an important point which calls for further research. Scholarship or scholastic aptitude being on the average high in the college with college entrance board examinations, it is possible that the left-handed individuals, if less well adjusted or less able to compete, for any reason, do not reach us, as we seem to have no maladjusted stutterers whose difficulty is definitely traceable to left-handedness, so far as the index and a rapid check on handedness in various performances indicates, when both the superior speech group, and all of the girls held for speech-correction in a single year, are studied.

### TABLE IV

Median scores on unimanual activities, as listed in inventory.

| | | | | | |
|---|---|---|---|---|---|
| RN | (Superior speech group) . | 50 | Range of scores . | 19–66 |
| CORR | (Corrective speech group) | 51 | Range of scores . | 29–66 |
| S | (Stutterers) . . . | 56 | Range of scores . | 29–60 |

Eliminating from the above scores those of the questionable LN cases listed as right-handed-changed, the scores run as follows :—

| | Median Scores | | Range |
|---|---|---|---|
| RN . . . . . | 51 | Range of scores . | 26–66 |
| CORR . . . . . | 51 | Range of scores . | 29–66 |
| S (no right-handed-changed | 56 | Range of scores . | 29–60 |
| or left-hand dominance found) | | | |

In the above table it will be seen that when we eliminate the doubtful cases of the two right-handed changed individuals, one from each group, we find the same median score for the 48 individuals remaining, or for the 24 composing each group, this median being 51 in each group. In spite of the speech defect, we find the median score for all stutterers in this year's entering class (4 students) to be 56, or several points higher than that found for the two equated groups. It would be unfair to draw other conclusions from these findings, due to the small number of cases represented, even though this small sampling happens to represent all of the stutterers found in the entering class in the Fall of 1931.

TABLE V

Percentage of R, L and X responses to handedness inventory for bimanual activities

| | R | L | X | Unans. |
|---|---|---|---|---|
| RN . | ·49 | ·36 | ·11 | ·04 |
| CORR . | ·48 | ·31 | ·09 | ·12 |
| S . | ·65 | ·25 | ·10 | ·00 |

The small number of unanswered questions in the superior speech or RN group is not sufficient to account for the difference in scores as only 4 per cent. were unanswered. Assuming that these should all be listed under " R ", the total percentage would still be below that found by Jasper,[1] as he finds 64 per cent. for his " RN " group, whereas we find 49 per cent. for our RN group, leaving a higher percentage of " L " and " X " responses than are found in Jasper's group.

The corrective group contains about the same number of " R " responses as does the superior (RN) group. The difference between the " L " and " X " responses is not great, and due to the groups being smaller than those

---

[1] Jasper, *op. cit.*, p. 77, Table II.

originally tested, may be considered negligible. The
12 per cent. of unanswered questions in this group might
have changed the results somewhat and may be significant,
from the very fact that the students felt unable to
answer them.

In the stutterers' group all questions were answered,
and we find a high percentage of responses under "right",
corresponding very closely to the percentage found by
Jasper for his RN (normal) group. The percentage under
" L " and " X " was in each case less than that found
for the corrective group as a whole or for the superior
speech group.

Our scores represent a much more restricted range
than those found by Jasper, and exact comparison is
impossible due to the difference in the composition of the
Iowa groups as compared with those available for our
tests. The number of stutterers found in this year's
group at Mount Holyoke is so small, and the indications
of left-dominance so slight, that additional tests beyond
those given would be necessary in order to establish the
fact of such dominance.

It seems possible that the scholarship factor may be
an important point to consider, and that the mere fact
of left-dominance may enter into the adjustment problem
of certain students, so that they tend to enter colleges
where the college entrance system is less severe. The
fact that there is evident in the two groups tested and in
the group of stutterers, no student who lists herself as
left-handed, and only two who are reported as " right-
handed-changed ",[1] makes it impossible to draw any
sweeping conclusions as to the difference in findings as
between the Iowa and the Mount Holyoke groups.

The inventory is useful in ascertaining the fact of
present handedness, and may be used as a basis for
further experimentation. In the case of stutterers, or
maladjusted individuals making a negative or a zero
score, it is helpful, as a check on the motor activities and
preferences of the individual, and in speech rehabilitation.

[1] Right-handed, having been changed from left to right.

The high median score obtained by the stutterers on the inventory compares favourably with the scholarship, as three out of four of these students are well above average in scholastic attainment.  The fourth, who is in the list of doubtful students, made a score of 60 on the inventory, showing positive right-handedness in her responses.

Of the two right-handed-changed (possibly LN students) both the one in the corrective group and the one in the superior speech group are below the average of this year's Freshman class in scholarship, one being in the lowest half, the other in the lowest tenth in the class, and the latter being in the speech-correction group.

Although interference with dominance, due to right-handed changed condition has not led to stuttering in either of these instances, it is a possible factor in the scholastic attainment and social adjustment, if we accept this evidence.

The inventory is intended for stutterers, rather than for corrective groups as a whole, but is useful in locating those whose dominance has been changed by educational procedures, earlier in life.  We do not find, in our groups, corrective, superior, and stutterers, the wide range of difference located by Travis and Jasper in the Iowa groups.  More extensive experiments would need to be undertaken, involving considerably more apparatus than is at present available in our laboratories in order to check in detail on absolute dominance.  We find the inventory useful as a part of the speech testing procedure, particularly in comparing a corrective speech group with a control or superior speech group, and in studying possible " dominance " indicators in any unselected group.

## SUMMARY

According to Travis and Jasper, the results for the right-handed control group should show cerebral dominance, by the left hemisphere.  The corrective group, and particularly the stutterers, should show wavering in different muscular patterns.  Moreover the control group should be consistent in hand, ear, muscle and eye dominance, whereas the corrective and stutter-groups should vary, and that variation be highly correlated with speech defects.

We do not find definite evidences of such dominance, or of such cleavages as between the control and corrective, or control and stutterers' groups.  We do find a higher percentage of left-hand responses in the S group as compared with the RN group, but we find fewer ambidextrous subjects in both the control and the stutterers' group.  We find a higher percentage of right-handedness in both groups than are given by Travis and Jasper (p. 77).

Summarizing the results of Table III for eye, ear, hand and muscle responses as checked by means of the activities in table, we find :—

Groups { Control / Corrective / Stutterers

| *Eye Preferences* | *Ear Preferences* | *Hand Preferences* |
|---|---|---|
| More rt. responses in RN group. | Rt. and L. dom. is equal in S group. | All right-handed now. |
| More left responses in corrective and stutterers' group. | Rt. and X dom. is equal in RN group. Higher percentage of CORR and S use either ear than in RN group. | 2 right-handed-changed but no stutterers. |

## MUSCLE PREFERENCES

Muscular dominance not greatly different as between groups.

   A. *Ball Throwing.*
      All groups right-handed.

   B. *Swing Bat.*
      RN group 1 L subject.
            1 X subject.
      CORR group all right.
      S group 1 X subject.
         (No signif. difference between groups.)

   C. *Shuffling Cards.*
      72 per cent. rt.-handed in RN group.
      75 per cent. rt.-handed in corrective group.
      50 per cent. rt.-handed (S group).
      50 per cent. ambidextrous (S group).
      (Results positive for S group.)

D. *Turning Pages.*

RN group 32 per cent. L or X answers.
CORR group 16 per cent. L answers.
S group 25 per cent. L answers.

(Results do not indicate more L or X
responses from the corrective or the
S groups.)

E. *Tennis Racquet.*

All 100 per cent. right-handed.

(Result does not favour handedness theory.)

This table indicates that dominance is not clear in the RN group, but is evenly divided between R and X responses. The responses from the group of stutterers are also evenly divided but between Rt. and Left preferences. Higher percentage of those in Corrective and S groups use either ear, than in the RN group.

As to eye preferences, there are some indications of interference in dominance here, which might bear out the theory, as we find more right preferences in the RN group, but more left preferences in the corrective and the stutterers' groups.

As to general "handedness" all report at present as right-handed, but two report themselves right-handed-changed. These two subjects are not stutterers however, although they are poorly adjusted students, having difficulty in scholarship. One is in the RN group and the other in the speech corrective group (for ineffective speech).

As to muscular preferences, there is no clearly defined difference between groups, on the basis of the inventory used and with the addition of simple clinical methods for checking on sighting, aiming, etc. In ball throwing all groups were decidedly right-handed. In swinging bat all of the corrective group were right-handed. In the RN group one subject gave an L response and in the S group one reported X, so that there was no significant difference between groups here. In shuffling cards there were slightly more right-handed subjects in the corrective group than in the RN group. The S group was equally divided between R and X responses. The results seem to be significant for the S group in this activity. On turning pages of book there were more L and X responses from the RN group than from the corrective or the S group. There is no evidence of poorer muscle responses in the Corrective and S groups than in the RN group, on this activity. In handling tennis racquet all groups report right-handedness, answers on this point not favouring the theory of dominance as applied to stutterers.

Were more elaborate apparatus to be employed and a larger number of subjects tested, evidences of dominance might be more clearly indicated. We have confined ourselves to the inventory and to such clinical tests as are frequently used for simple indications of right- or left-handedness, or dominance, as in sighting, aiming, measuring with the eye, listening with the ear, using certain muscle-sets, and handedness as based upon training from childhood.

The comparisons made by Travis and his associates are between groups of stutterers and non-stutterers, and it must be borne in mind that our groups were chiefly composed of non-stutterers, or speech-correctives other than stutterers, and a normal-speech group. Travis makes no claim for the theory of cerebral dominance as applied to forms of speech disorder other than stuttering, and the results for his groups and our own are not strictly comparable, therefore. Moreover, the training factors in handedness may have so overridden native tendencies that the earlier tendency towards left-handedness is not apparent in our college group, as it might have been with younger subjects. It was our purpose to ascertain whether the theory of cerebral dominance might be applied to speech defects other than stuttering. While we found some significant differences between the stutterers and non-stutterers in our groups, and between well-adjusted and poorly adjusted students, we did not find that the factor of dominance seemed to be important in determining differences between the normal speech group and the corrective group.

It may be, however, that as right-handed individuals

have developed a more varied use and skill of the right hand and arm, it is to be expected that the recorded response from this limb would exceed in speed that of the left arm and hand, without the necessity of any native unilateral dominance, and that just the opposite would be true of left-handed persons who have remained left-handed in manual activities.

### REFERENCE

" Neuromuscular Organization in Stutterers ", by Herbert H. Jasper, University of Iowa Studies in Psychology, No. XV, Psychol. Monog., Vol. XLIII, 1932, pp. 172–174. By courtesy of L. E. Travis, State University of Iowa.

### HANDEDNESS INDEX

Name ....................................................

Age .......................... Sex....................

Race................... Nationality....................

Are you right-handed or left-handed *now* ?....................

Were you ever changed from left- to right-handedness ?..........

Did you ever stutter ?.............. At what age ?..........
For how long ?..............

Did you ever have the right arm or hand injured for any length of time ?............ For how long ?...............
At what age ?..............

In using tools with long handles, the hands may be used in one of two ways :

A. Right hand near outer end of handle, left hand nearer the " business end " of the instrument—such as hoe, rake, etc.

B. Left hand near outer end of handle, right hand nearer the " business end " of the instrument.

If in using the following tools, you almost always use your hands as in " A ", draw a circle around " A ".

If you almost always use your hands as in " B ", draw a circle around " B ".

If you have no particular choice, draw a circle around " X ".

| | | | | | |
|---|---|---|---|---|---|
| 1. Hoe . | . | . A B X | 6. Spade | . | . A B X |
| 2. Rake . | . | . A B X | 7. Axe . | . | . A B X |
| 3. Pitchfork | . | . A B X | 8. Ball bat | . | . A B X |
| 4. Shovel | . | . A B X | 9. Golf club . | | . A B X |
| 5. Broom | . | . A B X | | | |

10. In which direction do you ordinarily sweep : (1) toward the right ; (2) toward the left ; (3) no particular choice ?

11. From which shoulder do you ordinarily swing a baseball bat : (1) right ; (2) left ; (3) no particular choice ?

In doing the following acts, one hand does all or almost all of the work. If you almost always use the right hand, draw a circle around " R ". If you almost always use the left hand, draw a circle around " L ". If you have no particular choice, or if you use both hands (as, for example, shaving one side of your face with one hand, and the other side with the other hand), draw a circle around " X ". Answer only for those acts which you have actually done.

1. Which hand drives billiard cue ? . . . . R L X
2. Which hand swings tennis racquet ? . . . R L X
3. Which hand throws a ball ? . . . . . R L X
4. With which foot do you kick ? . . . . R L X
5. Which foot steps on a spade ? . . . . R L X
6. Which hand does most in shuffling cards ? . . R L X
7. Which hand deals the cards ? . . . . R L X
8. Which hand works lever in filling your pen ? . . R L X
9. Which hand turns the pages as you read ? . . R L X
10. Which hand puts the letter in the envelope ? . R L X
11. Which hand puts the stamp on the envelope ? . R L X
12. Which hand tears open envelope ? . . . R L X
13. Which eye stays open when you aim a gun ? . . R L X
14. Against which shoulder do you hold butt of gun ? R L X
15. Which hand holds knife when you whittle ? . . R L X
16. Which hand cuts with the knife in eating ? . . R L X
17. Which hand holds the fork in eating ? . . . R L X
18. Which hand uses the salt shaker ? . . . R L X
19. (You hold a dish in one hand and wash or wipe it with the other.) Which hand washes the dish ? . R L X
20. Which hand wipes the dish ? . . . . R L X
21. Which hand combs your hair ? . . . . R L X
22. Which hand strops your razor ? . . . . R L X
23. Which hand shaves your face ? . . . . R L X
24. Which hand uses the powder-puff ? . . . R L X
25. Which hand uses the tooth-brush ? . . . R L X
26. Which hand winds your watch ? . . . . R L X
27. Which hand scratches matches ? . . . . R L X
28. Which hand holds your cigarette ? . . . R L X
29. Which hand uses the dust cloth ? . . . . R L X
30. Which hand uses the needle in sewing ? . . . R L X
31. Which hand holds the thread in threading the needle ? R L X
32. Which hand uses the scissors ? . . . . R L X
33. When you wash your hands, which hand rubs the soap on the other ? . . . . . . R L X
34. Which hand wraps the tie around when you tie your tie ? . . . . . . . . R L X
35. Which hand would you use for lifting and carrying a cup level full of water ? . . . . R L X
36. Which hand uses a saw ? . . . . . R L X
37. Which hand uses a hammer ? . . . . R L X
38. Which hand uses a screw-driver ? . . . . R L X
39. Which hand uses wrenches ? . . . . R L X
40. Which hand cranks a car ? . . . . . R L X

41. Which hand uses a key in a lock ? . . . R L X
42. Which hand turns nuts on bolts ? . . . . R L X
43. Which hand handles the money when you pay for
    something ? . . . . . . . R L X
44. Which side do you sleep on ? . . . . R L X
45. Which hand holds a paper cup for drinking ? . . R L X
46. In jumping which foot gives the last push ? . . R L X
47. Which hand goes in coat sleeve first ? . . . R L X
48. Under which arm do you usually carry books ? . R L X
49. Which hand turns a door knob ? . . . . R L X
50. Which hand holds the receiver when telephoning ? . R L X
51. Which hand usually pulls out a drawer ? . . R L X
52. Which hand hangs up your hat ? . . . . R L X
53. Which hand stirs when mixing things ? . . R L X
54. Which hand picks up right shoe when dressing ? . R L X
55. Which hand picks up left shoe when dressing ? . R L X
56. Which shoe do you take off first ? . . . R L X
57. Which shoe is put on first ? . . . . R L X
58. Which stocking do you put on first ? . . . R L X
59. Which stocking do you take off first ? . . . R L X
60. Which glove is put on first ? . . . . R L X
61. Which hand turns key when locking a door ? . . R L X
62. Which hand reaches to pick up small object on floor
    in front of you ? . . . . . . R L X
63. Which hand writes letters ? . . . . . R L X
64. Which hand draws pictures ? . . . . R L X
65. Which hand does figuring ? . . . . . R L X
66. Which hand erases on paper ? . . . . R L X
67. Which hand does the most manipulating when tying
    shoe string ? . . . . . . . R L X
68. Which hand leads in reaching to a high shelf ? . R L X
69. Which hand uses the can-opener ? . . . R L X
70. Which hand turns egg-beater ? . . . . R L X
71. Which hand turns on water-tap ? . . . . R L X
72. Which hand takes mail out of box ? . . . R L X
73. Which hand pulls corks from bottles ? . . . R L X
74. Which hand supports you in rising from sitting
    position on floor ? . . . . . . R L X
75. When standing with both feet together which foot
    goes forward first to catch yourself when you start
    to fall ? . . . . . . . . R L X
76. Which ear do you turn towards a sound that is hard
    to hear ? . . . . . . . . R L X

# CHAPTER XI

## ORAL AND SILENT READING

### *Introduction*

READING, as a school subject, formerly meant oral inter-pretation. Children were taught to articulate correctly, to follow certain rules of oratory or declamation with precision in enunciation and speech mechanics, paying little attention to comprehension and content of material read. Reading experiments conducted for the purpose of analysing the processes involved, have caused a shifting of emphasis from oral reading to silent perception, or reading for speed and comprehension.

Since the experiments of Pintner (1913) a number of investigators have been fostering this shift of emphasis, believing that schools have been spending too much time in oral and too little in silent reading, from the fourth grade upwards. Until a few years ago educators agreed that oral reading was superior to silent reading as an aid to comprehension, but recent investigation has shown that silent reading is more economical for the assimilation of ideas than is oral reading. Research indicates that when the chief emphasis is upon oral reading throughout the eight grades in the elementary schools, pupils frequently build up fixed ideas, wrong habits of pronunciation and motor eye movements associated with the reading process, and that all of these combine to slow down the reading rate, so that the child deals with his material in a very laborious fashion.[1,2]

Among the most important steps in reading enumerated by Starch [3] are the following :—

[1] O'Brien, *Reading, Its Psychology and Pedagogy*, 1926, pp. 25–139.

[2] Schmidt, W. A., " An Experimental Study in the Psychology of Reading ", Suppl., Educ. Monog., I, 2, April 1917.

[3] Starch, D., *Educa. Psychol.*, 1921, p. 260.

1. Receiving the visual stimuli from the printed page.

2. Range of field of distinct vision cast upon the retina.

3. Range of attention and apprehension of visual stimuli.

4. Eye movements.

5. Transmission of visual impressions from the retina to the visual centres of the brain.

6. Arousal of associations which aid in interpretation.

7. Transmission of impulses from the visual centres to the motor speech centres.

8. Transmission of motor speech impulses from speech centres to surface organs of speech.

9. Execution of movements of speech organs in speaking words.

Huey found that slow readers averaged 2·5 words per second in silent reading, whereas fast readers covered 9·8 words per second. Oral reading rate, according to Huey, averaged 2·2 words per second for slow readers, and 4·7 words per second for fast readers.[1] Becker, Erdmann and Dodge found that perception proceeded by word-wholes and phrases, and that fluctuation was absent.[2,3] Quantz [4] reported that rapid readers excelled in grasp of connected material and that there was a correlation between speed in reading and speed in comprehension.

Dearborn with a group of thirty subjects found that rapid readers read three times faster than slow readers.[5] Schmidt claimed [6] that one-fourth of the time in the elementary schools was devoted to the teaching of reading. Schmidt [6] found that the average number of pauses

[1] Huey, E. B., The Psychology and Pedagogy of Reading.

[2] Becker, " Experimentelle und kritische Beiträge zur Psychologie des Lesens bei kurzen Expositionszeiten ", Zeitschr. f. Psychol. und Physiol. der Sinnesorgane, Bd. 36, Hefte 1, u, 2, pp. 19–73.

[3] Erdmann and Dodge, Psychol. Untersuchungen über das Lesen auf Experimenteller Grundlage, 1898.

[4] Quantz, J. O., " Problems in the Psychology of Reading ", Psy. Rev. Monog. Sup., 2, 1.

[5] Dearborn, W. F., " Psychol. of Reading ", Columbia Univ. Contrib. to Philos. and Psychol., XIV, No. 1, 1906, p. 116 ff.

[6] Schmidt, W. A., " An Experimental Study in the Psychology of Reading ", Suppl., Educ. Monog., I, No. 2, April 1917.

per line varied from 4·1 to 10·8 per line for silent reading, and from 6·1 to 11·5 per line for oral reading. The average number of words perceived per pause in silent reading ranged from 2·15 to 0·93 words ; in oral reading the range was from 1·62 to 0·86 words. The rapid silent readers read more than twice as fast as the slowest silent readers.

Investigations into the psychology of reading, mastery of its mechanics and growth in reading ability show that the early laborious stage of reading is passed by some children in the second grade but that most children do not master the technique sufficiently to read easily until they reach the third grade. Once the mastery is attained, the rate seems to remain relatively constant.

It has been shown that motor adjustment aids in clearness of perception, as it is during the fixation pauses that recognition and perception take place. These arouse associations which lead to comprehension, analysis and synthesis of subject material.

Some of the most important studies of motor movements associated with reading are those of Dearborn, Cattell and Hamilton. Following Dearborn and Cattell at Columbia, Hamilton worked with the Cattell fall-screen and tachistoscope. He used short sentences, phrases and words, to compare reading abilities and to measure the amount read per exposure. He also studied the variations in amount read from exposure to exposure and the distribution of amounts read over the area of clear vision.[1] Typed reading material was exposed for ·021 seconds. The five subjects were, with one exception, trained psychologists.

His results for comprehension showed that sentences had a marked advantage over separate words or phrases, and that phrases had an advantage over separate words. He found that with all subjects there was 100 per cent. comprehension in reading sentences, whereas the range of comprehension for phrase reading was 71·5 per cent. to 90 per cent. in the five subjects. The variation in

[1] Hamilton, F. M., *Arch. of Psychol.*, 9, Dec. 1907, pp. 1–56.

Q

comprehension of words for all five subjects was 28·3 per cent. words to 55·2 per cent. words, or only 50 per cent. at most, as compared with comprehension when *sentences* were read.

## Causes of Reading Disability

Schmitt [1] traced the difficulty in learning to read to the child's inability to learn phonetics. Her pupils could not form associations between the form of the letters and their sounds. She concluded that phonetics, as generally taught in the class-room, do not adequately meet the needs of the slow reader or the non-reader in grades one and two. She also found evidence of psychopathic tendencies in many of her subjects and concluded that all children unable to acquire phonetics and to read intelligently are probably quite inefficient in forming associations between sounds and symbols, between words and meanings. She found the span of attention, power of perception and apprehension below average in all her subjects.

Fernald and Keller [2] find that children with reading disabilities are limited in visual, auditory, or kinæsthetic imagery, defective in speech or articulation, often left-handed and frequently subject to defective emotional control. Such children can be adequately trained only by special methods which strengthen the visual, auditory and kinæsthetic associations. They emphasize the importance of building up stronger kinæsthetic linkages between words, symbols and meanings by tracing or writing them as they are being read and pronounced. Not only are they able by these methods to secure improvement, but they cite cases in which public school pupils and university students have advanced from the poor scholarship group to the highest scholarship group

[1] Schmitt, C., " Congenital Word Blindness or Inability to Learn to Read ", *Elem. Sch. Jour.*, 18, 9, May 1918, and June 1918.

[2] Fernald, G. M., and Keller, H., " The Effect of Kinæsthetic Factors in the Development of Word Recognition in the Case of Non-Readers ", *Jour. of Educ. Research*, 1921.

within a few months following the beginning of special training in reading, writing and spelling by the Fernald method.

Among common causes of reading disability, the following are summarized from O'Brien, W. S. Gray, Dearborn, Schmidt, Starch, Huey and C. T. Gray:—[1]

1. Inferior mental endowment.
2. Poor auditory, visual or kinæsthetic memory.
3. Defective vision.
4. Limited span of recognition.
5. Congenital word blindness.
6. Ineffective motor adjustments, slow eye-movements, etc.
7. Lack of power of concentration and attention.
8. Poor vocabulary.
9. Inadequate training in phonetics.
10. Insufficient motivation.
11. Psychopathic tendencies.
12. Unfavourable physical conditions such as the presence of diseased glands, tonsils, adenoids, dental caries, defective nervous system.
13. Left-handedness.

Among remedies suggested the following are among the most important :—

1. Strengthening the bonds or associations between visual, auditory and kinæsthetic impressions.
2. Adequate training in phonetics.
3. Exercises in increased speed and accuracy of recognition.
4. Exercises to widen the span of recognition and to aid in interpretation.
5. Decreased vocalization during reading ; decreased accessory motor movements generally.

[1] References :
Gray, C. T., *Types of Reading Ability as Exhibited through Tests.*
O'Brien, *op. cit.*, p. 213.
Gray, W. S., " Value of Informal Tests of Reading Accomplishment ",
*Jour. of Educ. Research*, Feb. 1927.

6. Training to increase the power of analysis and comprehension of material read by frequent drills, checking up the child by making graphic records of results as a stimulus to his efforts.

7. Training in concentration and gain in power of attention to the task in hand.

8. Reading with a time limit.

Dearborn has recently suggested that left-handedness itself is not a cause. He holds that unilateral cerebral dominance, as indicated by left-handedness or by eye dominance may be the cause.[1]

## *College Reading*

Following various experiments with grade school children, educators began to turn their attention to the problem of reading in college. If it was possible for school pupils, under direction, to make great gains in rate and comprehension, would similar training insure greater skill in reading among college students ? It was commonly assumed that increase in speed and comprehension in reading might be closely linked up with scholastic attainment and academic standing. One of the most important studies made along this line was that of Eurich [2] at University of Minnesota, who attempted to measure comprehension, speed and accuracy in reading and vocabulary. A special reading test was devised (the Minnesota Reading Examination), and a Vocabulary Test was prepared. The results showed that there was a gain in vocabulary when the measuring paragraphs which were used duplicated or reproduced a part of the original material. There was no vocabulary transfer in general ; the student reacted to the specific training received, and the improvement was within the range of the previous training given.

[1] Dearborn, W. F., " Harvard Grad. School of Educ. Monographs ", Contrib. to Educa.

[2] Eurich, A. C., *The Reading Abilities of College Students*, Univ. of Minn. Press, 1931.

As a result of these experiments Eurich felt that in all fields taught in college students should receive special instruction to increase their special vocabularies. Since the Minnesota experiment extended over a period of only three to six months, the investigator felt that a longer and more intensive training period was needed for conclusive results.

Carroll in his experimental studies [1] found that the gain made by his practice groups was more than 100 per cent. greater than that of the control groups when the former received definite training in reading directions.

Headley [2] mentions the following as aids in reading for college students :—

(A) That the student endeavour to get as much as possible in a single act of comprehension ; that she increase the visual-perceptual span, enlarge her span of ideas and grasp more than one word at each fixation.

(B) Motivation must be found to create an urge to read well. Reading with a time limit is suggested with definite attempts to improve one's own time record.

He thought students should be able to read about 225 words of ordinary text-book material per minute.

Other suggestions include attention to the enlarging of one's vocabulary ; trying to grasp the plan of the author ; analysing material as read ; being an active agent oneself, by thinking as one reads ; supplementing in advance what the author has thought out. Material must be read and sifted as consumed.

Bird [3] finds that different college courses demand very unequal amounts of reading and that within a course the reading skill demanded varies from time to time. Some courses consist mostly of lecturing and laboratory work ;

[1] Carroll, *An Experimental Study of Comprehension in Reading,* Columbia Univ., 1926.

[2] Headley, *How to Study in College,* 1926, pp. 257–82.

[3] Bird, C., *Effective Study Habits,* 1931, pp. 97–126.

others emphasize the rapid assimilation of reading materials from many different sources. Rapid reading and comprehension are always an asset ; slow, laborious reading is a handicap. Some students in any entering class may surpass the reading average for seniors ; others are not up to the eighth grade level in skill in reading.

Arnold [1] found that 7 per cent. of a group of college students made silent reading scores below the eighth grade median in comprehension, and 30 per cent. made lower scores in speed of reading. In special reading tests given to all Freshmen at Ohio State University during a two-year period, Pressey [2] found that approximately 20 per cent. of Freshmen read less efficiently than the average eighth grade pupil. She also found that generally the students who tested low on standard reading tests did relatively poor work in courses where efficient reading was essential.[2]

Starch [3] reports that about one-fourth of university students read less rapidly than the average fifth grade pupil. In the University of Minnesota tests, less than half of the students made comprehension scores which equalled or exceeded the median score of high school seniors. The remainder scattered mostly within the range of high school students, but 6 per cent. fell below the eighth grade level. Very low scores on reading tests generally are found in students who have difficulty in understanding and in recalling the subject-matter of the various courses.

After using the Van Wagenen English Literature Scale A at the University of Minnesota with 272 college students, in " How to Study " classes, Bird [4] compared the results with standards for high school and eighth grade pupils.

---

[1] Arnold, H. J., *Disabilities of College Students in Certain " Tool Subjects "*, Phi Delta Kappan, 1929, 11, pp. 169–74.

[2] Pressey, L. C., " Training College Freshmen to Read ", Ohio College Association Bulletin, 55, p. 566.

[3] Starch, *Educational Psychology*, p. 186.

[4] Bird, C., *Effective Study Habits*, 1931, p. 99.

This is shown in the following table : [1]—

|  | Below Grade 8 | Grade 8 | Freshmen | Sophs. | Jrs. | Srs. |
|---|---|---|---|---|---|---|
| Median score college students | ? | 77 | 80 | 84 | 87 | 90 |
| Those reaching above standard | No. 16 Per cent. 5·9 | No. 15 Per cent. 5·5 | No. 30 Per cent. 11·0 | No. 34 Per cent. 12·5 | No. 48 Per cent. 17·6 | No. 129 Per cent. 47·5 |

Book [2] compared reading efficiency with scholastic attainment and found that among 673 students, those with a reading efficiency of 75 per cent. or above earned 32 credit points as compared with students of less than 20 per cent. efficiency, who earned about 11 credit points during the first semester.

Pressey [3] found that academic marks improved with increased efficiency in reading. Remedial training was given to the 422 students whose grades fell in the lowest 25 per cent. of the entering class at Ohio State University. Only 212 improved their reading sufficiently to equal the median reading score for all Freshmen. The average point-hour-ratio of the trained group was 1·97 in contrast to that of 1·46 for the control group. The author therefore stresses the importance of reading efficiency as a factor in scholarship.

### Studies of the Mechanics of Reading

An important study was made by Tinker,[4] of the interfixation points between pauses. He found that eye movements were not continuous, and that the only " sweeping glance " observed was of the passage of the eye from the end of one line to the beginning of another ;

[1] Bird, C., *Effective Study Habits*, 1931, p. 99.

[2] Book, W. F., " How Well College Students can Read ", *Sch. and Soc.*, 1927, 26, pp. 242–48.

[3] Pressey, Mrs. L. C., " Training College Freshmen to Read ", Ohio State University Bulletin, 55.

[4] Tinker, M. A., " Eye-Movement Duration, Pause Duration, and Reading Time ", *Psychol. Rev.*, 1928, 35, pp. 385–397.

the rest is a series of pauses or fixations. 94 per cent. of the time was occupied by fixations. During pauses words were found to be in the clearest field of vision and during this time comprehension occurred ; during left to right movements of the eye words were not perceived. Pauses vary in duration.

Buswell, in his experiments at the University of Chicago,[1] discovered that the eye moves in advance of the voice. The term eye-voice span has been applied to the distance between the word which is spoken and the word on which the eye fixates. This varies widely in different individuals. It is minimal in small children just learning to read, and optimal in mature readers. Good readers generally have a longer eye-voice span than poor readers. Buswell found that the average eye-voice span for good readers was 13·8 letter-spaces as compared with 8·7 letter-spaces for poor readers.

Tachistoscopic studies made by Dearborn and Cattell at Columbia University have already been mentioned.[2] Such studies show that eye movements are frequently regressive, i.e., retracings of material already read. The eyes move back leftwards to refixate. The causes of these movements seem to be unfamiliarity with subject-matter, poor vocabulary, lack of attention and meagre comprehension. The more the reader pronounces in inner speech the words as he reads, the more frequent are these regressions.

Brooks[3] found that interfixation time could be changed but little by practice. Reading speed and comprehension are partly indicated by the nature of the eye movements, and such movements thus become valuable aids in the diagnosis of reading disability.

Photographic studies indicate that some adults make as few as four pauses per line while others make as many

[1] Buswell, G. T., " An Experimental Study of the Eye-Voice Span in Reading ", Educ. Monog. Suppl., 17, Dec. 1920, Univ. of Chic. Press.

[2] Cattell, J. M., " Reactions and Perceptions ", Essays Philosoph. and Psychol. in Honour of William James.

[3] Brooks, F. D., The Appl. Psychol. of Reading, p. 278.

as fourteen, under the same conditions. Faulty eye movements are rarely the cause, but rather a symptom of poor reading. Attempts to overcome regressive movements of the eyes and to lengthen the perceptual span are often productive of good results. Emphasis should be centred, however, upon improvement in vocabulary, speed in reading and analytic thinking, rather than upon muscle movements.

Experimenters agree in stressing the value of reading with a time limit, and the avoidance of excessive vocalization, as lip movement and inner speech are slower than visual comprehension and the latter is actually retarded when it is accompanied by the former. Huey [1] found that the average rate of 20 students reading silently was 5·63 words per second at ordinary speed, and 8·21 per second at maximal speed. In reading aloud the rate was 3·55 per second at ordinary speed and 4·58 per second at maximal speed.

At the University of Indiana, Book also found great individual differences in the reading abilities of students. In his investigations in 1927 the best readers were seven times as good as the slow readers. There was also a steady decline in the number of " credit points " from best to poorest readers. After undertaking a " How to Study " course to improve reading rate and comprehension, with 54 students, these students gained 102 per cent. in one semester in these functions. [2]

Mount Holyoke investigators have also joined in the educational movement for the study of individual differences in reading. The problem of remedial measures in reading at Mount Holyoke College arose as a natural result of the tests in oral and silent reading given by the writer to all entering students in the Fall of each year from 1922 to 1931 in the Department of Psychology as a part of the required speech tests. The tests showed that there were each year a good many students of poor reading

[1] Huey, E. B., *The Psychology and Pedagogy of Reading.*
[2] Book, W. F., " How Well can the College Student Read ", *Sch. and Soc.*, V, 26, Aug. 20, 1927.

ability well below the median for their class on the material read. An apparent relationship between low scholarship and poor reading led to the belief that remedial reading measures might be advisable. Accordingly a faculty committee on reading was appointed and after a study of the reports presented, the following conclusions were reached :—

1. That there is a wide range in reading ability in each college Freshman class.

2. That the median rate for Mount Holyoke College Freshmen is somewhat above the median for the average adult.

3. That students who read slowly have approximately the same rate in oral and in silent reading.

4. That there may be some connection between reading rate and proficiency in speech, since many of the girls held for corrective speech are found to be in the lowest fourth of the class in rate of reading.

5. That although there is some gain in reading ability through the college years, a great range of ability is still present in the Junior year, as shown by re-tests of reading rate given to Sophomores and Juniors who were originally in the lowest one-fourth of the Freshman class.

6. That the median of the poorest readers in the Sophomore and Junior classes on Whipple's H.S. and College Reading Test is above the standard given by Book and Whipple for university Freshmen.

7. That the median grades received in college courses by our group of poor readers are below the median grades of their respective classes.

Assuming that poor reading might be a cause of poor scholarship, it was decided to carry on an experiment in the improvement of reading with a small number of students during the year 1928–29, and a small appropriation was made for that purpose. Miss Mary Ellen Hayes, a Major in Psychology who had already shown an active interest in this field, was chosen to work upon the problem during her Senior year under the writer and Prof. Herbert Moore.

This work has been reported in detail in an unpublished thesis filed at Mount Holyoke College entitled " Improving the Reading Rate of College Students ".[1]

## *The Experiment*

The aim of this study was to help girls who were having difficulty in reading, and to discover effective methods for improving reading rate and comprehension.

The students were limited to a small control group sent to us in response to a letter addressed to all heads of departments, requesting that they refer a limited number of students to the Psychology Department for special aid in reading. Girls whose poor grades or ineffective work were thought to be due to " lack of time ", " slow reading " and " backwardness " were suggested as those most in need of such remedial training.

Departments responded by sending a total of ten students. Six of them began work early in November of the college year. These constituted Class A. The remainder started work at the beginning of the second semester. These were called Class B.

The work was undertaken under difficulties. The girls were of unequal age, ability and interest. There was no compulsion used and they frequently neglected home assignments in reading, due to the pressure of their regular college work. No equivalent control group was provided.

## *Diagnosis*

A study of the Freshman reading test scores in oral and silent reading [2, 3] showed that in the silent reading test one student was well above the median for the class,

---

[1] Hayes, M. E., Dept. of Psychology Library, Mount Holyoke College, 1929.

*Diagnostic Tests.*

[2] Whipple, G., *Oral Reading Test.*

[3] Starch, D., *Silent Reading Test*, 9, Educational Psychology.

three were just at the median, three were slightly below and three very much below.

To obtain more recent information concerning present reading ability, the Whipple H.S. and College Reading Tests Form A were given.

The median scores are compared in the following table :—

TABLE I

| | |
|---|---|
| Average score for college Freshmen given by Whipple . . . . . . | 10·5 or 52·5 per cent. |
| Median score of 415 Freshman girls at University of Indiana (Book's study) . . | 10·65 or 53·16 per cent. |
| Median score of poorest readers, Mount Holyoke College Freshmen . . . . | 12 or 60 per cent. |
| Median score of special reading class, Mount Holyoke . . . . . . | 11 or 55 per cent. |
| Median score of six poorest students of reading group . . . . . . . | 9·5 or 47·5 per cent. |

This shows the median for the special training group to be below that for the poorest group of readers for the Freshman class but still above the median for Indiana University students. The six poorest students had scores indicating a definite reading handicap in comparison with other students in the same institution.

A study of the academic standing of these six special group students (Group A) yields the following information ; three cases of low scholastic attainment, one who is well above average in scholarship, the other two being usually the recipients of rather poor grades. It is significant that there seems to be some increase in reading ability in college, independent of training, as girls in the special group who came from Class of 1930 averaged highest, those from the Class of 1931 next highest, and those from the Class of 1932 (Sophomores) lowest in scholarship.

Members of the group were also compared to discover the relation of intelligence and college grades to reading. The student of highest scholarship in the group headed all three lists. Two students of low scholarship were at the foot of the lists for intelligence and reading ability.

Individual conferences were given to each student before group remedial measures were undertaken. These were both to reassure the student as to the meaning of the special work, and in order that the worker might understand the difficulty better.   The following items were discussed or noted :—

> General appearance and personality.
> Condition of health ; hygiene of the eyes.
> Attitude towards work ; discriminating, original imitative.
> Special interests, academic and extra-curricular.
> Ability to concentrate and to comprehend.
> Time-and-place study habits.
> Method of note-taking.
> Average number of pages per hour read.
> Special difficulties with reading.

Practically all students were desirous of improving their rate and comprehension in reading.  Some claimed that re-reading was always necessary in order to comprehend material covered.   Others found difficulty in condensing and taking notes ; most of them were not at all confident about picking out important points in assignments ;  concentration was found to be difficult ; distraction was frequent even in the quiet of the college library.   History and Economics were subjects most frequently mentioned in connection with reading difficulty, as these called for a great deal of supplementary reading in which " skimming " was often advisable.

The eye movements were only roughly studied, but it was found that in number of fixations and regressive movements the two girls having poorest scholarship were inferior to the rest of the group.

## Methods

The reading class met for one period a week from mid-November to mid-April.  Topics such as the following were discussed and special reading tests were prepared, covering some of the material used for discussion :—

*Samples of Topics*

The value of rapid reading.
The relation between rate and comprehension in reading.
Skimming and its use in reading.
Concentration and attention.
How to get important points in reading.
How to improve one's vocabulary.
How to keep mentally fit.
How to keep physically fit.
Learning and remembering.

*Daily Practice Exercises*

Each student was required to keep a daily record of reading without note-taking on one of her regular assignments, and to try to improve her rate. Each girl graphed her results as this stimulated her to improve her own record. The records varied with length of time spent, time of day, difficulty of material and other conditions. For several days before the December vacation each girl received daily in her mail-box an exercise in skimming. This consisted of two mimeographed pages to be read through hurriedly in order to find the one answer requested. Eight selections were devised for this purpose, matched as nearly as possible in length and difficulty. The first five were based upon Kitson's *How to Use Your Mind,* and the last three upon Headley's *How to Study in College.*

During the second semester a test was given each week. It consisted of three-page articles of approximately equal difficulty, all taken from Headley. At the end of each reading a true-false test of 11 statements was given, three minutes being allowed for reading as far as possible and one minute for taking the test. Two scores resulted : (1) the number of lines read, and (2) the number of true-false answers which were correct.

Just before the mid-year examinations a test was given on " How to take an Examination ". The subjects were asked to read and take notes on this assignment, and their notes were later analysed, graded and discussed.

In planning study time, each student was asked to report the number of hours per week spent in classes, laboratory and study.   There was considerable variation in the answers for the ten girls, the range being from 35 to 72 hours a week.   Economy of time would seem to be an important factor in budgeting a student's work effectively.

Whipple's H.S. and College Reading Test Form A was given at the first meeting and Form B at the last meeting of the class.

## *Results*

Without taking notes, students reading from Stone [1] improved from 770 to 870 lines read in a period of thirty minutes, showing a gain of 18 per cent.   With simpler material the rate in reading increased from 22 to 31 pages in thirty minutes, and in taking notes while reading in a Psychology text-book, the rate increased 77 per cent. or from 9 to 16 pages in thirty minutes.

One girl at the foot of the group at the outset, improved 50 per cent. in reading rate in one week.   A second student who stood near the foot of the group improved 54 per cent. in a single week.   At one time or another five of the students showed good improvement in their daily practice. The remaining students were near the upper end of the group at the outset.

In skimming exercises there was general improvement from the first to the last exercise.   The curves were irregular, however, as one would expect with non-standardized tests devised for the occasion.   Although all of the material came from two books (Kitson and Headley) they were probably not all of equal difficulty.

In the weekly tests for rate and comprehension the group which worked throughout the year made the most progress.   There was a general trend of improvement for both groups A and B, some individuals progressing more rapidly than others.   The true-false questions merely served to warn the girl that she must understand what

---

[1] Stone, C., *Oral and Silent Reading*.

she was reading.    Comprehension did not seem to be diminished by reading for speed.    This agrees with the findings of Stone [1] that speed may be increased without damage to comprehension if the emphasis is placed mainly on speed with only a brief check-up for comprehension.

Improvement in rate alone with the Whipple Test Form A amounted to 46 per cent.    The score was the number of words read per minute.

A questionnaire was given to each student to find out which exercises she considered most valuable and which seemed to have benefited her most.    The students reported that the work was of especial value to them in such studies as Economics, Religion, Philosophy, History and English.    Gain in power of concentration, ability to skim assignments and realization of the value of conscious effort were mentioned as perhaps the most important results.

Among the topics discussed in the readings, the following were mentioned as especially helpful :—

> Practice in skimming.
> Concentration.
> True-false tests.
> Graphing one's improvement in reading.
> Budgeting one's time.
> The value of rapid reading.
> Environmental conditions for study.
> Attitude towards work.
> Purpose in reading.
> Individual conferences.

All students felt that the work in the special reading class should be more definitely correlated with their regular work.

### Summary

1. Not all of the students in the special group were below the median for their class in reading ability, but none were markedly fast readers.

[1] Stone, C., *Oral and Silent Reading.*

2. A relation was found between academic records, reading efficiency and scholastic attainment. If this holds true of larger groups also, those low in scholastic attainment or in academic averages might benefit greatly from improvement in their reading habits.

3. The most effective elements during the weekly training periods were :—

    (1) Motivation through conscious effort for improvement.

    (2) Practice in skimming.

4. The most effective devices for recording weekly practices were :—

    (1) Cutting the work to half-hour periods.

    (2) Keeping a record of the pages read.

    (3) Using the same book.

    (4) Keeping notes of environmental conditions.

    (5) Reading without taking notes.

5. In this experiment every student felt that she had benefited by the discussion and exercises, and showed definite improvement in reading ability, based on the tests.

6. The average improvement shown in the Whipple Form A test was 46 per cent. in rate alone and 18 per cent. in rate and comprehension combined.

### Oral and Silent Reading Tests for Freshmen

During the analysis of speech tests given to all entering students in the fall of the year at Mount Holyoke College in the years 1922 to 1925, it was observed by the writer that there were wide variations in reading rate among college freshmen. Some were well below the median for their class, and others below the eighth grade median for silent reading. Since certain fundamental processes involved in reading are rather closely linked up with the speech reactions, it seemed worth while to make a more careful analysis of the results of the tests in oral and

R

silent reading, which had extended over a considerable period of years.

Beginning with the class entering in the Fall of 1925, the writer made a study of the rates in oral and silent reading, reporting to the English department those students who were found to be in the highest fourth of the class, and those who were in the lowest fourth of the class in both tests, together with a separate report for each test. The median for the class was calculated and a graph of the class results for reading was prepared.

Book [1] in his studies at the University of Indiana had already reported that he found some graduate students who were 17·1 times as good as the poorest. The best students made a score of 19 out of 20 points on assignments in reading, while the poorest made a score of 1 out of 20 points.

We found each year in the group of girls held for speech-correction, a number who were in the lowest fourth of the class in silent reading rate or in both oral and silent reading rates. Several of these students were also in the low scholarship group.

The material for graphs of the results for the years 1925 to 1931, was obtained through the use of Whipple's standardized test [2] for oral reading, and Starch's test for silent reading.[3] In giving these tests at the University of Wisconsin in 1920–22 the writer had found the median for oral reading to be three words per second or 180 words per minute. The median on this material at Mount Holyoke for the seven years 1925–31 was 180 words per minute with a range of 58 to 393 words per minute. Some students read orally 6·7 times as fast as others, under identical conditions.

In silent reading at Wisconsin, the median for a group of university students was four words per second or 240 words per minute. The median at Mount Holyoke

[1] Book, W. F., How Well can College Students Read ?  *Sch. and Soc.*, Aug. 1927.

[2] Whipple, *Plain Prose Test for Oral Reading*, No. 77281–A.

[3] Starch, D., *Silent Reading Test No. 9*, No. 17049, Speech Testing Material.

during the seven-year period was 310 words per minute, with a range of 82 to 609 words per minute. This indicates that some girls were reading silently 7·4 times as fast as others under identical conditions. The writer tested several faculty members also, and none of them read less than 10 words per second, or at the rate of 600 words per minute. This raised an interesting question. Were reading assignments in courses made on the basis of the more rapid reading rate of members of the faculty, or on the basis of the average reading rate of college students ? We have not yet discovered a satisfactory answer to this question, but it has led to an appreciation by our teachers of the need for considering variations in reading rate, in making assignments.

Rapid skimming of assignments of medium difficulty is estimated to be at the rate of about 400 words per minute. Each year we have found many girls who could not read as rapidly as this.

It may be seen from the Table of Cumulative Frequencies for the entire period that 697 students are below the median range of 178–201 for the class in oral or in silent reading.

## Summary

One hundred and four students or about $5\frac{1}{2}$ per cent. made scores representing the lowest fourth in silent reading rate (58 to 195 words per minute). About twenty-five students or 1·33 per cent. made scores representing the lowest fourth in oral reading rate. Six hundred and ninety-seven students or 37 per cent. of total are below the median in oral reading, and nine hundred and twenty-eight students or 49 per cent. are below the median in silent reading rate.

In the Fall of 1927, thirty students in an entering class of 289 were in the lowest group in both oral and silent reading rates, while twenty-five students were highest in both. One-third of the girls selected for speech-correction that year were in the lowest fourth of the class in both oral and silent reading rates.

In January 1928, a re-test was given to the sophomores and juniors who in their freshman year had been in the lowest fourth of the class in silent reading. This included twenty-two sophomores and forty-four juniors. There were some unavoidable absences so that the entire group of those who stood in the lowest fourth was not tested, but these constitute a majority.

The range for these sophomores in their freshman year had been 124–244 words per minute. In January their range was 106–512 words per minute, showing that while some had improved considerably, there were others who had not improved in speed in reading during the year and a half. The median range for this group had been 202–225 words per minute in freshman year, and had in sophomore year improved to 274–297 words per minute.

For the juniors re-tested, the range (freshman year) had been 130–226 words per minute. In January of the junior year the rate had improved to 222–489 words per minute or double that of freshman year for some students, and faster for all of them than in freshman year. The median for the group in September of their freshman year had been 220–225 words per minute, and in the junior year it was 298–321 words per minute, i.e. well above the median for the freshman year.

As to inequalities within the group it was found that some still read five times as fast as others. In the class as a whole in freshman year, there were students who read seven times as fast as others.

Even by the junior year, the performance of those originally in the lowest group without special training had not equalled that of the better readers of the class in their freshman year.

What were some of the causes of this slow reading ? We suggest as factors a low level of attention, defective vision, lack of judgment, poor memory, slow eye movements, length of eye-voice span, regressive movements of the eyes and movements of the lips or inner speech while reading. Watson [1] identifies thought with inaudible

---

[1] Watson, J., *Psychol. from the Standpoint of the Behaviourist.*

speech.  Woodworth [1] takes exception to this point of view.  It is obvious that there is some relationship between reading rate and fluency or speed in making motor-speech adjustments.  If the general motor efficiency of the individual is slow or sluggish, may it not be that the motor-speech impulses in skilled performances like reading and speaking also are retarded in transmission to the peripheral speech mechanism in the case of the slow reader ?  These students seem to need special training in reading, skimming, perceiving readily and reproducing material.  Speed in reading may possibly improve speed in speaking or even speed in forming judgment, and keenness of perceptual ability.  The speech and eye movements are so closely related in learning to read, write and speak, that slow performance in one seems closely linked with ineffective performance in the others.

If emphasis is placed primarily on reading for speed and comprehension, fluency of speech may not be improved.  Inner speech and motor lip movements with silent reading certainly slow down the process and interfere with speed of perception.  Exercises in silent reading for speed and comprehension, with a brief oral test on the material, is valuable to slow readers, as it trains them to read observantly, knowing that they will be checked up, while relieving them from the necessity of looking for minute details.  This may train them to analyse the material as they read, so as to be prepared to reproduce the gist of the assignment.  Incidentally it may train them in oral speech, ease and fluency in utterance, if discussions of material read follow the silent reading assignment.

Chart I is a composite of the curves for the seven years 1925–1931.  When the annual graphs were plotted we were surprised to find such great similarity between the curves.  In no single year does the curve deviate markedly from the average for all seven years (Chart I).  The median and range for each year are very close to those for the whole period.  This seems to indicate that

[1] Woodworth, R., *Psychology*, 1930, Rev. Edit.

if preparatory schools are making any special effort towards remedial reading, either for speed or comprehension, the results do not show in our tests. Within the seven years involved, improved methods in reading have apparently not affected the preparatory schools to any appreciable extent.

In silent reading the difference ranged from about 100 to 600 words per minute. Slow readers cover material only one-sixth as fast as fast readers. In the group of slow readers approximately 5·8 per cent., or about 18 girls in each freshman class of about 275 girls, tend to fall below the eighth grade level.

During the college year 1931–1932, a major in Psychology, Miss Eunice Russell, was assigned the problem of analysing the reading curves for freshmen, for the past seven years. A study of the composite graphs has been given in the Table of Cumulative Frequencies, Table I, and separate results for oral and silent reading have been given in Charts II and III. Both curves are presented in Chart I. Results of this study of slow reading indicate : (1) That superfluous motor movements are associated with reading, many of which seem to be a carry-over of infantile habits, such as biting the nails, clenching the fist, scowling, squinting and the like. (2) That there is a tendency among many of the slow readers to employ lip movements in reading or to use inner speech. Such students should practise reading by visual recognition and with an endeavour to eliminate as far as possible the motor representations, reducing vocalization and articulation to a minimum. (3) That regressive and slow eye movements are frequent. The eye instead of moving progressively forward, regresses, or refixates frequently, slowing up the comprehension of new material, and causing long pauses at the fixation points. Headley believes that poor vocabulary is responsible for a good many of the regressive movements in reading.

Many slow readers have not learned to vary the amount of attention to suit the material read. Rapid skimming of newspapers, novels and magazines seems never to have occurred to them as they had not realized that such reading should require less time than the reading of technical books and more important literature within their field of special interest.

These hints for reading after Lyman, are usually recommended to these plodding readers who have never acquired the ability to skim material :—

1. What is the author's main idea ?  Keep this idea in mind.

2. Weigh the various parts in relation to the main idea, discarding the least important parts.

3. Vary the reading rate according to purpose and material.

4. Read deliberately with special attention to essential parts.  To this we suggest marking your own books and making brief notes to aid in fixing the main ideas. Motivation and interest are two other very important factors.

### Conclusion

In conclusion we call attention to Stone's three classes of slow readers and his suggestions for the improvement of each, as we have found that the difficulties which he suggests are common in college.

*First :* There are the non-readers found in the early grades of the elementary schools, who have made little progress along academic lines.  Here special methods are used to diagnose the child's difficulty, to arouse an interest, and to apply the methods most needed in the individual case.  This type of student does not usually reach the college, although some cases diagnosed as word-blindness appear, which closely resemble the non-reader child in many ways.  In college we find more frequently readers who are up to the median in oral reading rate, but who are slow and careless in silent reading with poor comprehension.

*Second :* We have the good oral readers who are careless in silent reading.  These students need to develop a factual and experiential background for reading and should check themselves up both in concentration and in comprehension.[1]

*Third :* We have those who are slow in reading. These students should establish regular movements of the eyes, develop rapid recognition of words and increase the eye-voice span by direct effort. They must direct their attention to content and cultivate the ability to skim material, setting for themselves a time limit.

The following is an outline of the remedial work done with a fourth grade child referred to our Psychology Department. The case was diagnosed by Miss Hayes under the supervision of the department, and the remedial work was carried out by Miss Elizabeth Carr, another major in Psychology working upon the problem of remedial reading.

### Remedial Reading, Case A [2]

A. was a ten-year-old child in the fourth grade retarded in school because of her difficulty in learning to read. Her I.Q. on the Stanford-Binet scale was 85. On the Pressey Primary Classification Test (Form A) she made a score of 53, the median for third grade in this test being 56. She was given the Seguin Test, the Two-Figure and the Five-Figure Form Board Tests, the Healy Mare-Foal Test and the Knox Cube Test. In all of these she measured below the average for her age and grade.

She was given the reading tests of the following type in October, soon after she was referred, receiving scores as follows :—

| Test | | Oct. | Jan. (1930) (Scores) | Norms for Grade 4 |
|---|---|---|---|---|
| Burgess Silent Reading Test PS1 | . . | 22 | 32 | 50 |
| Monroe Silent Reading Test : | | | | |
| | Rate . . . | 74 | 73 | 121 |
| | Comprehension . | 3 | 4 | 7·7 |
| Haggerty Sigma Test 1 | . . . . | 2 | 9 | 18 |
| Test 2 | . . . . | 4 | 7 | 20 |
| Curtis Tests : | | | | |
| | Words. . . | 77 | 86 | 145 |
| | Questions . . | 19 | 27 | 30 |
| | Compreh. Index . | 36 | 31 | 89 |
| Gray Oral R. Test . | . . . . | 40 | 41 | 47 |

[1] Gray, p. 10, Case 5.

[2] Carr, Elizabeth, *Remedial Work in Reading,* unpublished paper in Dept. of Psychology, Jan. 1930.

*Remedial Measures*

After being tested, she came twice each week for a short training period. Speed in reading was one of the first things in which she was drilled. She was first asked to read for ten minutes and then counted the number of lines she had read, so she could record her progress on a graph. The material used was Little Black Sambo, His Baby Elephant, and the Tale of Mrs. Tubbs. Her comprehension of this material was very poor as she seemed to pay little attention to content. Even when the purpose of this reading was explained to her and she was instructed to be prepared to answer questions on the material, she was unable to do so.

Attention was then directed to the improvement of comprehension. She was given short stories to read, consisting of only two or three pages in good type or fairly large print. These were sometimes read orally and sometimes silently. She was asked for a résumé of each story after reading. As stories were selected which were within her range of interest, she soon showed improvement in understanding, and the assignments were gradually lengthened. Although her speed in reading gradually increased and her comprehension improved between October and January of the school year, she was still five points below the norm on comprehension in the Curtis Reading Test after her three months of training.

The words missed in reading were drilled upon by the Fernald kinæsthetic method. Words learned one day were repeated the next day, and if she could spell them she was allowed to write them in her note-book under new words learned. In two months she learned to spell correctly twenty-two new words. In spelling she tended to write down all of the letters of the word, with but little attention to the correct order. This difficulty was lessened by having her analyse the words more carefully from a phonetic standpoint, and to learn to write the word so that the symbols appeared in their proper sequence, pronouncing the syllables as she wrote.

Other devices were used such as matching the names of objects with pictures; filling in blanks in sentences; following typewritten directions; tagging objects with their correct names; building up sentences by using separate printed words. Easy reading and grasp of content were the aims of the instructor while seeking to increase both speed and comprehension. It was found necessary to continue the work into the second semester of the year in order to aid the child sufficiently to enable her to advance with her grade in school, the ordinary instruction in reading in the school-room not being sufficiently suited to her needs.

Additional educational measures have been worked out during the year 1931–32 by psychology majors, working with non-reader children in the local schools. These have been reported upon in detail in the unpublished theses submitted for honours work by Miss Martha Town and Miss Margaret Meader, in the department of psychology.

Miss Meader followed the more recent trend of analysing " comprehension abilities " into the various factors of which it is composed. She then endeavoured to improve these factors in individual cases, and to speed up the reading rate in each.

Miss Town's work contained a number of original and successful devices for engaging the interest and concentration of the non-reader child, and her methods are especially worthy of attention because of the results which she was able to secure by their application to the children with whom she worked.

## Conclusion

Reading is the act of perusing and of interpreting that which is written. According to the psychologist [1] there are certain bodily accompaniments of attention which are important in comprehending printed symbols. Nervous excitation may influence the act of attention favourably or unfavourably. If antagonistic impulses occur simul-

[1] Titchener, *Textbook of Psychology*, N.Y., 1909, pp. 299–301.

taneously, they may prevent the occurrence of any reaction by inhibiting the process through interference. Wundt postulated a special centre within the frontal lobes of the cortex which he believed served to control the inhibitory processes.   More recent theories teach that the control of inhibition and facilitation may involve the entire cortex, or that it may be diffused through several centres.   Some hold that when a sensation is clearly defined it is due to local excitation of a certain cortical centre, and that when the sensation is vague, poorly defined and obscure, it is of diffused cortical origin.[1]

We know that when right adjustments are acquired by children in the early learning stages of reading they are not easily displaced by defective and laborious habits. Many children, however, employ a great many extraneous muscle movements in reading, and they do so quite unconsciously.   Many small children in learning to read and write, as in learning to walk, protrude the tongue as though this organ served as an active agent in the mastery of hand and eye movements.   Whispering and use of the vocal organs frequently accompany the observation of words and pictures.   It is not recommended, however, as it slows up the reading rate, yet we find college students and others who have carried this habit over into maturity.

CORRELATIONS BETWEEN ORAL READING RATE

AND { SCHOLASTIC AVERAGE,
STANDING IN SCHOLASTIC APTITUDE (PSYCHOLOGICAL) TEST,
RATE IN SPONTANEOUS SPEECH

*Oral Reading and Spontaneous Speech Rate*

As the relationship between rate in oral reading and intelligence, scholarship and rate in spontaneous speech is largely a matter of conjecture in dealing with normal individuals, it was felt that a study of the coefficients of

[1] Titchener, *Textbook of Psychology*, N.Y., 1909, pp. 299–301.

correlation between these factors might be advisable. First we undertook to find out what relationship, if any, exists between rate in oral reading and rate in spontaneous speech. Using the Dvorak Correlation Chart [1] the scores of entering students for the classes of 1932 to 1935, consisting of 1083 students, were correlated. The relationship was less than one might have anticipated, although there was a slightly positive trend as the results were $r = +\cdot112$ (P.E. ± ·0299). Below are given the medians for the four years for this group of students ; according to the intervals by which the correlations were computed :—

|  |  | Medians |
|---|---|---|
| Spontaneous Speech Rate | . | 125–144 words per minute. |
| Oral Reading Rate | . . | 180–194 words per minute. |
|  |  | Mode |
| Spontaneous Speech Rate | . | 125–144 words per minute. |
| Oral Reading Rate | . . | 180–194 words per minute. |

Total number of students, 1083.

We find that the largest number of frequencies corresponded to the median range or central tendency for the group, in spontaneous speech rate, and in rate in oral reading, and there are indications that there is a slight positive correlation although the coefficient of correlation is small.

*Oral Reading and Scholarship Average,*
*for highest 10 per cent. in Oral Reading Rate*

Coefficients of correlation between oral reading rate and scholarship standing of girls who were in highest 10 per cent. of classes, in oral reading rate, each year 1925 to 1931 inclusive (seven years) :—

| Year 1925 | 1926 | 1927 | 1928 | 1929 | 1930 | 1931 |
|---|---|---|---|---|---|---|
| −·22 | −·09 | +·13 | −·17 | −·04 | +·11 | +·18 |

Calculation of the correlation between oral reading and scholarship for the above groups combined gave a coefficient $r = +\cdot049$ (P.E. ± ·052).

[1] Dvorak, *Correlation Chart,* 1930.

*Correlation between Oral Reading Rate and Scholastic Aptitude Tests for highest 10 per cent. of class in Oral Reading Rate.*

| Year 1925 | 1926 | 1927 | 1928 | 1929 | 1930 | 1931 |
|---|---|---|---|---|---|---|
| −·25 | +·19 | +·05 | −·20 | −·07 | −·07 | −·08 |

Correlating the oral reading with the scholastic aptitude standing for the whole seven years combined we find a coefficient of correlation of $r = -·067$ (P.E. ± ·055) or a negative correlation.

This leads us to ask whether some other factors might not give increased speed in reading to girls of low standing in the scholastic aptitude test. There are evidently a good many of the girls of average scholarship and ability who read at a rate which is above the median for the class, but rapid oral reading is not, according to these findings, highly correlated with scholarship standing, and in some cases our psychological rating scale gives indications of neurotic tendencies such as is sometimes shown in pathological speech, in cluttering and dysrhythmia, or in extreme nervousness. These fairly rapid readers frequently do not stand near the top of the scholarship list, nor do they appear in the topmost group in psychological rating. Good speech is apparently that which is associated more closely with an average rate of reading. It might be worth while to study girls whose scores were close to the median to see whether a relationship exists between a moderate rate of speech, and one which stands neither at the top nor at the foot of the scores for speed of oral reading.

The scores for the girls who stood in the lowest 10 per cent. of the class in oral reading were correlated, oral reading rate being compared with scholarship and scholastic aptitude scores.

The results were as follows :—

*Oral Reading and Scholarship Average*
*of lowest 10 per cent. of class in Oral Reading*

| Year 1925 | 1926 | 1927 | 1928 | 1929 | 1930 | 1931 |
|---|---|---|---|---|---|---|
| +·23 | +·05 | −·01 | +·06 | +·17 | −·06 | +·25 |

Correlating Oral Reading with Scholarship for the entire seven years we find that $r = + \cdot 258$ with P.E. of $\pm \cdot 048$.

The scores for students in oral reading rate who were in the lowest 10 per cent. of the class in this test were correlated with scholastic aptitude (psychological examination) with the following results :—

*Oral Reading Rate and Scholastic Aptitude, for those who were in lowest 10 per cent. of class in Oral Reading*

| Year 1925 | 1926 | 1927 | 1928 | 1929 | 1930 | 1931 |
|-----------|------|------|------|------|------|------|
| $- \cdot 05$ | $+ \cdot 03$ | $+ \cdot 26$ | $+ \cdot 24$ | $+ \cdot 28$ | $+ \cdot 24$ | $- \cdot 21$ |

The correlation for Oral Reading with the combined results of the scores in Scholastic Aptitude Test for the seven years gave the following coefficient :—

$$r = - \cdot 07$$
$$P.E. \pm \cdot 056$$

The result is rather surprising inasmuch as the results for several of the separate years gave indication of a slight positive tendency. (See years 1927–1930.)

There seems to be some relationship between the low scores in oral reading and scholarship, as the coefficient for the combined scores for seven years yields an $r$ of $+ \cdot 258$ (P.E. $\pm \cdot 048$). We find no such relationship, however, when oral reading rate for the lowest tenth of these classes is compared with the psychological rating, as in the table above.

*Summary*

There seems to be some positive relationship between low scores in oral reading and scholastic attainment. Between low scores and psychological rating we find no such relationship. Our findings when we compare oral reading for those who stood in the highest tenth of the classes in this performance, with scholarship average and with psychological rating were negative or indicated no close relationship.

There is evidence of a slight positive relationship between rate in oral reading and fluency or speed in utterance but the two seem not to be closely related.

## TABLE I

### ORAL AND SILENT READING TESTS

Class of 1929 to Class of 1935 inclusive
Fall 1925 to Fall 1931

MOUNT HOLYOKE COLLEGE

| | ORAL READING | | | SILENT READING | | |
|---|---|---|---|---|---|---|
| Words per Minute | Number of Students | Cumulative Frequency | Cumulative Percentage of Students | Number of Students | Cumulative Frequency | Cumulative Percentage of Students |
| 58–81 | 1 | 1 | ·05 | — | — | — |
| 82–105 | 14 | 15 | ·8 | 2 | 2 | ·1 |
| 106–129 | 10 | 25 | 1·33 | 9 | 11 | ·58 |
| 130–153 | 63 | 88 | 4·67 | 15 | 26 | 1·38 |
| 154–177 | 609 | 697 | 37·02 | 30 | 56 | 2·97 |
| *178–201 | 747 | 1444 | 76·69 | 48 | 104 | 5·52 |
| 202–225 | 358 | 1802 | 95·7 | 171 | 275 | 14·6 |
| 226–249 | 64 | 1866 | 99·1 | 154 | 429 | 22·78 |
| 250–273 | 10 | 1876 | 99·6 | 224 | 653 | 34·68 |
| 274–297 | 7 | 1883 | 100·00 | 275 | 928 | 49·28 |
| †298–321 | — | — | — | 268 | 1196 | 63·52 |
| 322–345 | — | — | — | 188 | 1384 | 73·5 |
| 346–369 | — | — | — | 154 | 1538 | 81·68 |
| 370–393 | — | — | — | 104 | 1642 | 87·2 |
| 394–417 | — | — | — | 76 | 1718 | 91·24 |
| 418–441 | — | — | — | 58 | 1776 | 94·32 |
| 442–465 | — | — | — | 27 | 1803 | 95·75 |
| 466–489 | — | — | — | 42 | 1845 | 97·98 |
| 490–513 | — | — | — | 18 | 1863 | 98·94 |
| 514–537 | — | — | — | 4 | 1867 | 99·15 |
| 538–561 | — | — | — | 3 | 1870 | 99·31 |
| 562–585 | — | — | — | 1 | 1871 | 99·36 |
| 586–609 | — | — | — | 12 | 1883 | 100·00 |

* Median for Oral Reading.      † Median for Silent Reading.

Number of students, 1883.

## TABLE II

### TABLE SHOWING MEDIANS FOR EACH SEPARATE YEAR IN ORAL READING RATE WITH STANDARD DEVIATIONS

| Year 1931 | | 1930 | | 1929 | | 1928 | | 1927 | | 1926 | | 1925 | |
|---|---|---|---|---|---|---|---|---|---|---|---|---|---|
| Med. 186 | S.D. ±31·79 | Med. 190 | S.D. ±19·86 | Med. 178 | S.D. ±19·34 | Med. 177 | S.D. ±21·53 | Med. 185 | S.D. ±24·98 | Med. 186 | S.D. ±24·21 | Med. 184 | S.D. ±18·45 |

Average S.D. 22·88.

Median for all classes in Oral Reading, 178–201 words per minute.

Material—Whipple Plain Prose Test.

I.  CHART SHOWING DISTRIBUTION OF SCORES IN ORAL
AND SILENT READING TESTS

(Years 1925–1931 inclusive)

MOUNT HOLYOKE COLLEGE FRESHMEN

(Number of Subjects—1883)

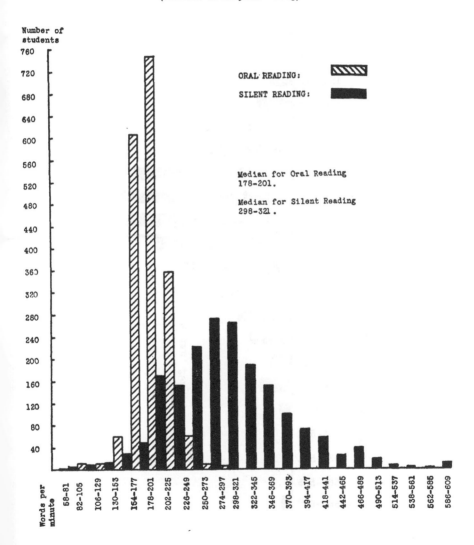

Number of
students

ORAL READING:

SILENT READING:

Median for Oral Reading
178–201.

Median for Silent Reading
298–321.

Words per
minute

S

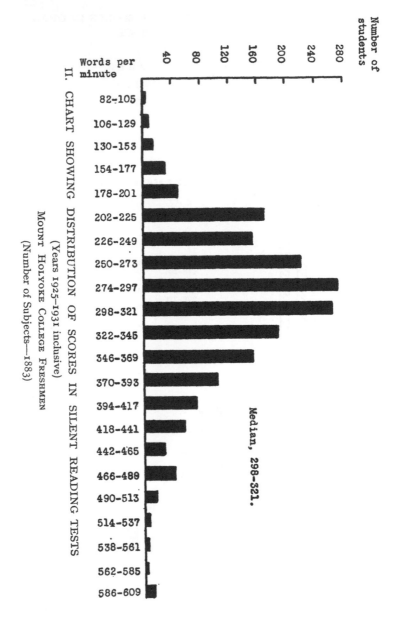

II. CHART SHOWING DISTRIBUTION OF SCORES IN SILENT READING TESTS
(Years 1925–1931 inclusive)
MOUNT HOLYOKE COLLEGE FRESHMEN
(Number of Subjects—1883)

III.  CHART SHOWING DISTRIBUTION OF SCORES IN
ORAL READING TESTS
(Years 1925–1931 inclusive)
MOUNT HOLYOKE COLLEGE FRESHMEN
(Number of Subjects—1883)

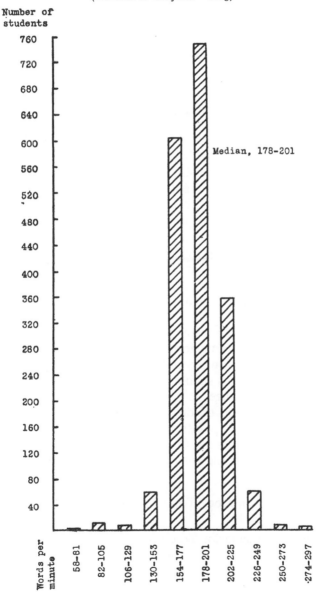

Median, 178-201

# CHAPTER XII

RESULTS OF SPEECH TESTS

*A*. NORMS FOR 3581 STUDENTS TESTED, 1920–31

*B*. CLASSIFICATION OF SPEECH LIMITATIONS

## *Nature of Tests*

THE tests used for ten years at Mount Holyoke College were the Blanton-Stinchfield Speech Measurements, devised at the University of Wisconsin, 1920–22, in order to provide some way of measuring school and university students as to speech attainment, and to enable the examiner to classify them as to speech proficiency or to place them in groups for class or individual training.

The measurements are divided into two parts, subjective judgment or off-hand estimate of the individual's performance being arranged for, and a series of objective measurements given, to which numerical values may be assigned.

The subjective measurements enable the examiner to estimate the student's performance as to behaviour, personality, social adjustment and general attitudes, and as to vocal characteristics such as quality, pitch, volume and distinctness of utterance.

The student is then graded on a scale of one to three, on each of the seven points included, making a possible total score of 21 points for this part of the test.

The objective measurements also include seven parts, viz. :—

Test I. Articulation Test A (consisting of all the sounds of English).

Test II. Articulation Test B (consonant combinations).

276

Test III. Oral Reading Rate (raw score, words per minute).

Test IV. Silent Reading Rate (raw score, words per minute).

Test V. Rate in Spontaneous Speech (raw score, words per minute).

Test VI. Percentage of relevant words (used in spontaneous speech).

Test VII. Vocabulary Score (number of words in 100 defined).

The original tests were given to a sufficient number of students to obtain temporary norms and correlation indexes, and in order that the more significant tests might be weighted for use in a team of tests to which numerical values might be given by the examiner. Since the working out of the original tests, additional score sheets have been added, on which the numerical computations may be omitted when the examiner wishes only the speech diagnosis and a rapid estimate of speech performance.

Temporary norms were established by the writer as the result of two studies made in Wisconsin, the first being the speech testing of 276 children Grades I to VIII in the Madison, Wisconsin Schools, and the other being a study of 151 university students, containing a speech corrective group and a control group. The norms have been published elsewhere.[1]

As tests involving reading ability offer some difficulty in giving speech tests in the early grades, a series of pictures containing the sounds listed by the International Phonetic Association, in its list of English sounds, was devised to replace sentences or words such as are contained in the tests given from Grades IV to VIII. This enables the examiner to secure the child's habitual speech

[1] " Formulation and Standardization of a Series of Graded Speech Tests ", Psychol. Monog. Series, Vol. 33, No. 2, 1923, p. 54.

Blanton-Stinchfield, *Speech Measurements, Manual*, No. 46087₅ C. H. Stoelting Co., Chicago, Ill., 1926, p. 14.

*Speech Tests and Their Uses*, p. 472 ; *A Programme of Speech Education in a Democracy*, p. 595.

reaction to the sounds in English by using a picture stimulus, when desired, and avoids the reading difficulty.

It was also found advisable to prepare a set of objects for use with pre-school children and for handicapped children such as blind, deaf, or mentally deficient children. These were first worked out by using the tests with a group of blind children at Perkins Institution for the Blind, in Boston. The results justified the opinion of the writer that a group of objects which would be suitable for use with blind children, and which were common enough so as to be rarely mistaken, would do equally well for normal pre-school children, for handicapped children such as deaf or crippled children, and for mentally deficient children. The continued use of these tests in speech clinics and in the Belchertown State School for the Feeble-minded has justified these conclusions.

### Speech Tests

During the years 1922–31, additional speech tests have been given to 290 children in Massachusetts grade schools as well as to one preparatory school group. The medians found, number of subjects and results are given in Table II.

### Comparison with Results of Earlier Tests

We find that the median for the larger number of Grade I children tested in Massachusetts is not quite so high as for the Madison group, the median in the Madison group being exactly 96 for 36 children, while for the Massachusetts group, the median falls between 93 and 95·5 on the above table. However, there is no great difference between the two, and this range between the medians probably lies close to what we shall find when a larger number of children have been tested, or approximately 93–96 on the Articulation Test A for all English sounds. This means that the average child in Grade I ought not to have difficulty with more than four to seven sounds, out of 100 test sounds given.

Articulation Test B was not used in Grades I and II.

## TABLE I
### TEMPORARY NORMS FOR A TEAM OF SPEECH TESTS
### MIDDLE GROUP SCORES

Name of Tests

| Grade | Artic. Test A Score | Artic. Test B Score | Oral R. Rate (Words per min.) | Silent R. Rate (per min.) | Rate in Spontaneous Sp. (per min.) | Per cent of Relevant Words used in Spont. Sp. | Vocab. | Age Norm. |
|---|---|---|---|---|---|---|---|---|
| I. | 96 | (not given) | (picture charts used for early grades) | — | 108–120 | 90–96 | 6 (in terms of use) | 6 (in terms of use) |
| II. | 96 | (not given) | | — | 108–120 | 90–96 | 6 (in terms of use) | 7 (in terms of use) |
| III. | 96 | 93–97 | 104–174 | 138–225 | 108–120 | 90–96 | 29–30 | 8 |
| IV. | 96 | 93–97 | 104–174 | 138–225 | 108–120 | 90–96 | 29–30 | 9 |
| V. | 96 | 93–97 | 104–174 | 138–225 | 108–120 | 90–96 | 47–48 | 10 |
| VI. | 96 | 93–97 | 104–174 | 138–225 | 120–150 | 90–96 | 47–48 | 11 |
| VII. | 96 | 93–97 | 104–174 | 138–225 | 120–150 | 90–96 | 50–53 | 12 |
| VIII. | 97 | 93–97 | 180–276 | 138–255 | 120–150 | 90–96 | 60— | 13–14 |
| University unselected group, 40 | 97·5 | 97·5 | | 204–258 | 120–150 | 96 | 73·5 (Terman adult norm, 65) (Superior adult norm, 75) | — |
| University selected group speech cases | 93 | 94 | 186 | 204–258 | 120–150 | 93 | 72 | — |

Temporary norms obtained by testing all pupils in each of eight grades (Madison, Wisconsin, Public Schools, 276 subjects). It also includes 151 university students, Wisconsin, making a total of 427 subjects tested, 1920–1922.

## TABLE II

Medians for Speech Tests given to Three Groups of Massachusetts School Children and to One Preparatory or High School Group, 1922–31

| Grades [1] | Artic. Test A | Artic. Test B | Oral R. | Silent R. | Rate in Spontan. Sp. | Per cent. Relevant Words | Vocab. | No. of Subjects |
|---|---|---|---|---|---|---|---|---|
| Grade I | 93–95½ | omitted | 28–72 | 22–96 | 74–100 | 96–97 | 6 words in terms of use | 87 |
| Grade II | 92 | ,, | 96 | — | — | — | — | 30 |
| Grade III | 96 | ,, | omitted | — | — | — | — | 27 |
| Grade IV | 94 | ,, | 120 | — | — | — | — | 33 |
| Grade V | 95 | ,, | 130 | — | — | — | — | 28 |
| Grade VI | 94 | ,, | 124 | — | — | — | — | 34 |
| Grade VII | 93 | ,, | 109 | — | — | — | — | 25 |
| Barrington School (High School Age) | 95 | 95–96 | 204 | 312–316 | 114 | 92 | 67 | 26 |
| | | | | | | Total Number of Subjects | | 290 |

[1] Grade I represents 87 children from three schools, South Hadley Centre, Woodlawn and Chicopee Falls Schools. Grades II-VII are medians for the tests in articulation and oral reading, given to the Woodlawn School children. The Preparatory School group represents 29 subjects from the Barrington School, a preparatory school for girls. All of the tests were given in Grade I and in the Barrington School, but for rapid diagnostic purposes and to keep within the time requirements, the tests were abbreviated when given in Grades II-VII in the Woodlawn School, it being possible to classify the speech defectives without giving the entire team of tests.

## Oral Reading Rate

The oral reading tests for Grades I and II were not given in the original testing at Madison, because of the reading difficulty involved, and the time element. The scores as given to 87 subjects in Massachusetts in Grade I, however, vary widely in range, the median for this grade lying between 28 and 72 words per minute, on the Gray Reading material for Grade I.

## Silent Reading Tests

The silent reading tests were omitted from the Madison team of tests, also, because of time element and reading difficulty, but were given to 87 Massachusetts children as shown in Table II. The variation in range should be noted for this grade, as the median was between 22 and 96 words per minute, or representing considerable difference in time, between the slow and fast readers. The range for the entire class was even greater than is shown by these medians, and the results for both oral and silent reading in these grades indicate that these children, some of them at least, require special assistance aside from that given during the regular reading period. Remedial reading is being given in both the Woodlawn and South Hadley Schools at the present time, the slow readers showing improvement under special direction, to date.

## Rate in Spontaneous Speech

The median for the Massachusetts group of 87 children was 74 to 100 words per minute, or slightly slower than that found for the Madison group of 36 first-grade children. A range of 74 to 120 is probably a fairer expression of what is to be expected of a larger group, since the medians for the two groups range from 74 to 120 words per minute as shown in Tables I and II.

*Percentage of Relevant Words*

The median for the Massachusetts group of 87 children was higher on this test than for the Madison children. The range for the medians of these two groups when compared, show that 90 to 97 per cent. relevant words were found when both groups were examined. (Tables I and II.)

*Vocabulary*

The Terman test is rather difficult for most children in Grade I, and all that they were asked to do was to define 6 words in terms of use. The median for the Massachusetts group of 87 children in this test was 6, as was also the median for the Madison Group.

*Articulation Test A.   Grades II to VII*

The median scores on this test Grades II to VII varied from 92–96, running slightly lower than the Madison group, on about the same number of children, in the Woodlawn School. The median for this test seems to lie between 92 and 96, according to these results for Grades II to VII.

*The Oral Reading Tests*

Median scores for Gray Oral Reading Test, Grades II to VII, ranged from 96 to 130, but if Grade II is omitted in order to compare the results for Grades III to VII in the Massachusetts group with those found for the Madison group, we find the range is 109–130 or still somewhat lower than the medians for the Madison group of about the same number of subjects. The difference in number tested is not great enough in these grades to account for the higher median found for the Madison group. There were 166 children in Grades III to VII in the Madison group, and 147 in the Massachusetts groups for these grades. When a larger number have been tested therefore we shall probably find that the range of 104 to 174, as given in Table I, is nearer the norm than that found in Table II for the Massachusetts group.

*Preparatory or High School Speech Tests*

For testing a group of 26 girls representing practically all of the girls then in attendance at the Barrington School, the Adult Speech Tests were used, as at present we know of no similar speech tests designed exclusively for high school use, aside from the Gray and Starch Reading Tests. The entire team of tests was given in order to compare the medians with those already found for college students.

The medians for Articulation Tests A and B are slightly lower than the median found for all Freshmen girls tested at Mount Holyoke College during the years 1922–31. The median for oral reading rate with this group was 204, or close to the college median of 208 found for a control group of college girls, years 1927–31.

The silent reading median in the preparatory school group was between 312 and 316, or close to the median found for the Mount Holyoke control group of 130 girls of normal speech, years 1927–31, whose median was 314 in this test.

The rate in Spontaneous Speech for the Barrington group was 114 words per minute, as compared with that for the Mount Holyoke control group of 130 girls, whose median was 137 words per minute. Both are within the range found for the original tests, however, at Wisconsin, the medians in Table I showing that the median for the Wisconsin group of unselected students was 120–150 words per minute in spontaneous speech.

The percentage of relevant words used in Spontaneous Speech in the Barrington group was 92 per cent. (median), and that for the Mount Holyoke control group of 130 girls was 96. The Wisconsin tentative norms on this test also give 96 as the median per cent. for relevant words (Table I).

The Vocabulary median for the Barrington group was 67 words in 100 defined. This is two points above Terman's norms for the civilian population, as he gives 65 for average adults, and 75 for superior adults. The

TABLE III

Revised Norms based upon Tests of 427 Subjects, Wisconsin, 290 Grade School and Preparatory School Subjects, Massachusetts, 2864 Students at Mount Holyoke College.  Total, 3581 Subjects.  Years 1920–31

| Grade | Artic. Test A | Artic. Test B | Oral R. Rate | Silent R. Rate | Spontaneous Speech | Per cent. Relevant Words | Vocabulary | Median Age |
|---|---|---|---|---|---|---|---|---|
| I. | 93–96 | Omitted | 28–72 | 22–96 | 74–120 | 90–97 | 6 words in terms of use | 6–1 |
| II. | 92–96 | ,, | 96 | omitted | 108–120 | 90–96 | 6 words in terms of use | 7–6 |
| III. | 92–96 | 93–97 | 104–174 | 138–225 | 108–120 | 90–96 | 29–30 | 8–5 |
| IV. | 92–96 | 93–97 | 104–174 | 138–225 | 108–120 | 90–96 | 29–30 | 9–6 |
| V. | 92–96 | 93–97 | 104–174 | 138–225 | 108–120 | 90–96 | 47–48 | 11–2 |
| VI. | 92–96 | 93–97 | 104–174 | 138–225 | 120–150 | 90–96 | 47–48 | 12–3 |
| VII. | 92–96 | 93–97 | 104–174 | 138–225 | 120–150 | 90–96 | 50–53 | 12–9–12–10 |
| VIII. | 97 | 93–97 | 104–174 | 138–255 | 120–150 | 90–96 | 60 | 14–1 |
| Preparatory or High School | 95 | 95–96 | 204 | 312–316 | 114 | 92 | 67 | 16 (Range 13–19 years) |
| College and University unselected groups of 2904 students | 96–97 | 98–100 | 170–276 | 204–340 | 120–150 | 96 | 73–78 | 18 (Range 16–22 years) |

Mount Holyoke control group median was 76·5 or higher than Terman's norm and higher than that found for the Barrington Preparatory school group.

The revised norms are based upon the study of 276 tests given in grades at Madison, Wisconsin, and 290 given in grades and preparatory schools in Massachusetts, or a total of 566 subjects for Grades I to VIII and high school. The adult or college tests were given to 151 subjects at the University of Wisconsin and to 2864 students at Mount Holyoke College, or 3015 college students tested, 1920 to 1931. This gives a total of 3581 speech tests given under the supervision of the writer.

TABLE IV

Norms for Adult Speech Test as given to 2864 Mount Holyoke College Students 1922–1931 (included in College Norms for Table III)

Median Scores

| Artic. Test A | Test B | Oral R. Rate | Silent R. Rate | Spontan. Sp. Rate | Per cent. Relevant Words | Vocab-ulary |
|---|---|---|---|---|---|---|
| 96–97 | 98–100 | 170–190 | 220–340 | 120–150 | 96 | 73–78 |

*Tentative Age Norms.*[1]

TABLE V

| Grade | Median Age | Age Range in Grade | No. of Subjects |
|---|---|---|---|
| I. | 6 yrs.–1 mo. | 5 yrs. to 8 yrs.–1 mo. | 61 |
| II. | 7–6 | 6–2 to 10–4 | 67 |
| III. | 8–5 | 7–1 to 11 yrs. | 55 |
| IV. | 9–6 | 8 to 13 yrs. | 68 |
| V. | 11–2 | 9–9 to 14–2 | 50 |
| VI. | 12–3 | 10–4 to 16–3 | 57 |
| VII, | 12–9 to 12–10 | 11–1 to 15–7 | 42 |
| VIII. | 14–1 | 12–4 to 15–8 | 39 |
| | | Total | 439 |

[1] Grades I to VII inclusive represent medians and age ranges for all of the grade children tested in the Madison, Wisconsin Schools and in the Woodlawn School, Massachusetts. Grade VIII was given only for the Madison Schools, there being no eighth grade in schools where the Massachusetts tests were given.

## ILLUSTRATIVE MATERIAL FROM THE SPEECH TEST

### Notice Regarding Freshman Speech Tests

*(Please read before you begin taking the tests)*

The speech tests which you are now taking, serve two purposes : first, they give each of you an opportunity to show something of the measure of your attainment in speech arts or interpretative work, if you have had previous training in any form of public speaking, dramatics, and the like ; and second, they enable us to place you in the particular speech group which may be most helpful to you now, and ultimately of the most service to you, as speech has an important bearing upon one's economic and social successes everywhere. It is important to make the most of it, because one must use one's native tongue constantly, whereas one may employ other languages only occasionally.

Not all colleges place an emphasis upon this important phase of personality development, but Mount Holyoke is anxious that its students should understand the principles of correct speech and enunciation sufficiently well to improve their speech during the time they are in the college, and by forming a definite speech standard, serve also as a good speech model in any community.

In about a week you will be notified as to your speech group, and Freshman class work in speech will not start until the class list has been posted upon the Speech Bulletin Board in the Post Office Corridor, following the sending out of the notices. As you will be later informed, you will be in one of the following speech groups :

Group I. Individual speech conferences, Freshman year.

Group II. Freshman Speech Class.

Group III. Girls placed in this group may defer their speech work until Sophomore, Junior, or Senior year, but it must be taken some time during the course for all except students entering with advanced standing in speech, due to work in some other college.

A few advanced students are excused on the basis of credit offered from other institutions. After you have taken the work to which you are assigned, you are free to elect speech courses.

Students preferring to elect the three-hour Course in Speech, may take this instead of the requirements in Groups II or III.

*This sheet is used when the examiner wishes to work out a speech index by using weighted
scores and doing the necessary computations.   There is a similar sheet for merely
recording the raw scores, if preferred, and in case the examiner does not wish to
use the computations included here.*

BLANTON-STINCHFIELD SPEECH MEASUREMENTS
COMPLETE SPEECH MEASUREMENT RATING SHEET [1]

For No. 5

Name.................................... Nationality....................................

Grade...................... Age........................ Sex......................

Address ........................................................................................

Measurements upper costal deflated....................inflated........................Vital

Capacity (spirometer).....................c.c.

## PART I. SUBJECTIVE MEASUREMENTS

| Maximum Points for Each Part. | | Examiner's Estimate Maximum 21 Points. |
|---|---|---|

### GENERAL BEHAVIOUR

(Grade on a scale of 1 to 3 ; 1 equals poor ; 2 average ; 3 very good)

1. 1–3 pts. A. Judge for control and activity (under or over-reacts)   ..................
2. 1–3 pts. B. Judge for specialized muscle movements, such as frowning, sprawling, extraneous muscle movements, tics, stuttering, etc.                    ..................
   C. Also judge for posture, physical anomalies, such as winging scapulæ, protuberant abdomen, depressed torso
3. 1–3 pts. D. Judge for poise, social adjustment, over-compensation, repression, anxiety, etc.                 ..................

### VOICE

4. 1–3 pts.  Judge for quality ; resonance, harsh, hoarse, nasal   ..................
5. 1–3 pts.  Judge for pitch ; range, inflection, very high or very low pitched tones                    ..................
6. 1–3 pts.  Judge for volume ; loudness, softness, medium, breathy, aspirate, etc.                    ..................
7. 1–3 pts.  Judge for distinctness and accuracy in articulation   ..................
   (Total number of possible points, 21)          Score A  ..................

## PART II. OBJECTIVE MEASUREMENTS

| | | | |
|---|---|---|---|
| Test I | Score in Articulation Test A. | . . | Multiplied by 5 .................. |
| Test II | Score in Articulation Test B. | . . | Multiplied by 7 .................. |
| Test III | Score in Oral Reading Rate . | . . | Multiplied by 3 .................. |
| | (Number of words per minute) | | |
| Test IV | Score in Silent Reading Rate | . . | Multiplied by 3 .................. |
| | (Number of words per minute) | | |
| Test V | Score for Rate in Spontaneous Speech . | | Multiplied by 2 .................. |
| | (Number of words per minute) | | |
| Test VI | Percentage of relevant words used in Spontaneous Speech | . . . | Multiplied by 50 .................. |
| Test VII | Vocabulary Score | . . . . | Multiplied by 10 .................. |
| | (Number of words in 100 defined) | | |

Total Score    ..................
Subtract             6950
Divide by 100 ..................
Speech Index   ..................
(Score B)

Score on Examiner's estimate and objective measurements are usually
approximately the same

[1] Courtesy, C. H. Stoelting & Co., Chicago (Copyrighted).

TABLE VI

Zero Coefficients, Unweighted, showing Relationship between Scores of Pupils in Different Grades and the Criterion (Subjective Speech Rating) in a Team of Seven Tests

276 Grade School Children, 40 Unselected College Students, 111 Speech-corrective Students, or a Total of 427 Subjects, Madison, Wisconsin.[1]

Subjective Rating and—

| | Test A | Test B | Rate in Spontan. Speech | Rate in Oral Reading | Rate in Silent Reading | Per cent. of Relevant Words | Vocab. | No. of Cases |
|---|---|---|---|---|---|---|---|---|
| Grade I. | ·62 | Omitted | ·05 | — | — | ·22 | ·23 | 36 |
| Grade II. | ·50 | ,, | ·10 | — | — | ·17 | ·13 | 38 |
| Grade III. | ·34 | ·15 | ·27 | ·487 | ·17 | ·016 | ·16 | 39 |
| Grade IV. | ·099 | ·19 | -·05 | ·53 | ·53 | ·27 | ·44 | 38 |
| Grade V. | ·26 | ·41 | ·62 | ·38 | ·35 | ·42 | ·16 | 39 |
| Grade VI. | ·09 | ·003 | ·061 | ·05 | ·05 | ·20 | ·39 | 28 |
| Grade VII. | ·56 | ·56 | ·33 | ·51 | ·63 | ·22 | ·25 | 22 |
| Grade VIII. | ·34 | ·43 | -·27 | ·22 | ·33 | ·56 | ·15 | 36 |
| University unselected group | ·385 | ·251 | ·258 | ·211 | ·588 | ·494 | ·428 | 40 |
| University selected group 111 speech-correction cases | ·64 | ·457 | ·308 | ·334 | ·369 | ·391 | ·34 | 111 |

The multiple correlation found from working the regression equation was ·731, or the maximum correlation that one may obtain from the team of tests and subjective rating, after they have been weighted to their optimum value.[1]

[1] Pp. 38-46. "The Formulation and Standardization of a Series of Graded Speech Tests", S. M. Stinchfield, Psychol. Monog., XXXIII, 2, 1923, Princeton, N.J.

TABLE VIb

MOUNT HOLYOKE COLLEGE GROUP, 1922 AND 1923

Zero Coefficients, Unweighted, showing Relationship between Scores of College Students and the Criterion (Subjective Speech Rating) in a Team of Seven Tests, 390 Students

| Year | Test A | Test B | Rate in Spontaneous Speech | Rate in Oral Reading | Rate in Silent Reading | Per cent. of Relevant Words | Vocabulary | No. of Cases |
|---|---|---|---|---|---|---|---|---|
| 1922 · · · | ·37 | ·39 | ·38 | ·22 | ·49 | ·27 | ·19 | 65 |
| 1923 · · · | ·18 | ·12 | ·27 | ·64 | ·11 | ·04 | ·31 | 325 |
| | | | | | | | Total | 390 |

The results of the tests at Mount Holyoke during the two years give a positive plus correlation on Articulation Tests A and B, Spontaneous Speech, Oral Reading, Silent Reading, and Vocabulary. These results compare favourably with those obtained for the University Unselected Group. On Percentage of Relevant Words, year 1923, there was a zero correlation. The correlations on this group of 390 students seem to indicate that there is a relationship between the criterion and the team of tests sufficiently high to warrant their continued use.

T

In the Fall of 1926 a comparison was made between the median scores assigned for each part of the speech tests, to a group of 82 students, consisting of 41 students from the speech corrective group for that year, and 41 students from a superior speech group. The results have been discussed elsewhere in detail and in order to compare those results with a similar rating made in the Fall of 1931 we will give only the average of the medians obtained for the speech tests and for the Seashore Musical Tests given in that year.

### TABLE VI

Rating in Speech Measurements and in Tests for Musical Talent, 1926

Number of students, Corrective Speech Group   .   41
Number of students, Superior Speech Group   .   41

Total   .   82 subjects

Median score obtained for a team of seven tests, for subjective estimate and speech index on objective measurements

|  | Superior Speech Group | Corrective Speech Group |
|---|---|---|
| Average of Medians . . . . . | 111·0 | 106·6 |
| Average of scores on Seashore Music Test . | C | C – |

In the above tests the objective performance of the superior speech group was higher than that of the corrective group on the Articulation Test, in Silent and Oral Reading rate and in Percentage of Relevant Words used in spontaneous speech. Sense of pitch, sense of intensity and tonal memory were somewhat less for the corrective group than for the superior group, indicating that the auditory discrimination is found to be less in the corrective group, and pointing to the fact already mentioned by Travis and others, that auditory discrimination is an important factor in the detection of correct speech sounds and plays an important part in the formation of correct habits of speech.[1]

It was felt that a study of a larger group might show important differences in both the medians for the speech tests and for the Seashore Music Tests, and so they were

[1] Travis, L. E., " The Relation between Faulty Speech and Lack of Certain Musical Talents ", Psychol. Monog., Vol. XXXVI, 10.

given to a group of 141 students held for speech correction, years 1927–1931 inclusive, and to a control group of students from an unselected group not held for speech correction, and consisting of 130 students. This made a total of 271 examined from five different classes, years 1927–1931. The results are given in detail as follows :—

### TABLE VII

Rating in Speech Measurements and in Tests for Musical Talent, 1927–31

Number of students in Corrective Groups    .    .    .    . 141
Number of unselected students from Better Speech Groups    . 130

Total .  271

| Median Scores | Control Better Speech Group | Corrective Speech Group |
|---|---|---|
| Speech median on subjective estimate    . | 16 | 14 |
| Speech index on objective measurements    . | 16 | 14 |
| Articulation Test A (all English sounds)    . | 97 | 93 |
| Articulation Test B (consonant combinations).    .    .    .    .    . | 98 | 92 |
| Oral Reading (words per minute)    .    . | 208 | 174·5 |
| Silent Reading (words per minute)    .    . | 314 | 280·5 |
| Spontaneous speech rate (words per minute) | 137 | 129·5 |
| Percentage relevant words    .    .    . | 96 | 95 |
| Vocabulary (words in 100 defined)    .    . | 76·5 | 74 |
| Average of medians    . | 117·6 | 107·5 |

Comparing the medians for the speech tests only, we find that when a larger group is tested the median for the corrective group in speech attainment is below that of a superior speech group, or for a group of unselected students having no speech difficulties. There is a surprising correspondence also between the scores obtained for the five-year group, as compared with the one-year group tested earlier on these functions.

Scores on Seashore Music Tests for two groups of students

Number of subjects in Speech Correction Group, 1931–32 .    . 33
Number of subjects in Psychology Course 101, year 1931–32    . 48
(both Freshman Groups)

Total subjects .    . 81

| Medians of Raw Scores (R.S.—Raw Score) | Pitch | Intensity | Time | Consonance | Average |
|---|---|---|---|---|---|
| Median-Freshman R.S.    . | . 80·04 | 88·54 | 75·23 | 69·29 | 78·28 |
| Median-Correctives R.S. . | . 79·27 | 84·12 | 75·09 | 65·27 | 75·91 |
| Difference between scores | . 0·77 | 4·42 | 0·14 | 4·02 | 2·29 |

The above comparison shows that the difference between these groups is greater in Intensity and Consonance than in Pitch and Time Discrimination. The difference in Pitch Discrimination between the two groups is less than in the one tested in 1926, at which time the corrective group median was lower in pitch, intensity and tonal memory than for the better speech group. We believe that the make-up of the group in this instance explains this difference, as the students used for a control group above were the total number of students in a Freshman Psychology Class, excluding any who were held for speech correction during that year. Had a superior speech group been used, rather than an unselected, non-corrective group, we believe that the difference in pitch discrimination would have appeared to be much greater in the corrective group. As it is, the corrective median is lower by a slight amount at least, in all four factors, including Pitch, Intensity, Time and Consonance Discrimination. The difference between the corrective and the superior speech and unselected groups of students is enough to warrant training and to be considered by the speech worker. We have found that in the corrective group, those who tested low on pitch discrimination during the past ten years, have very frequently been lispers, or those with blurred enunciation, who seemed incapable of distinguishing between a normal *s* and *z* sound, and a blurred sound which sometimes was actually a letter substitution, such as a *th* for an *s* or *z*. In such cases a voiced *th* was usually substituted for the voiced *z* sound, and the voiceless *th* for the voiceless *s* sound.

The possibility of high-frequency deafness for *s* and *z* sounds, particularly for *s*, has been mentioned by other investigators, particularly by English writers. A detailed study of such high-frequency deafness, by laboratory methods, would, we believe, yield important results.

The speech index on the objective measurements is often less than that found by the examiner's subjective or off-hand judgment of a girl, as girls often present a better appearance than is borne out in their actual speech performance.  The contradiction between appearance and performance may be used by the examiner, after the tests have been given, to show students just how much they need to improve in speech, in order to come up to the standard which the examiner feels is within the range of their possible attainment.  Personality and presentable appearance, combined with good speech, are certainly more favourable assets than one without the other.

On the other hand, many girls of high scholarship level make a very poor impression on the examiner when they first appear for the speech tests, and when such girls make a high objective score on the measurements such as oral and silent reading, vocabulary and spontaneous speech, they are told that they should try to develop personality and effective speech, as well as to develop the mental side, during their college days, since much will be expected of them, as a result of their mental acumen, and that they should therefore endeavour to bring their speech and personality reactions up to a more effective level, before they are graduated from college.

It is found that the girl of " average " attainment as rated by the examiner has a score very closely corresponding to her actual performance on the objective measurements.

In order to ascertain whether there were any important differences in the mental level of the corrective and non-corrective groups, the scores of the girls held for speech correction, years 1927–1931, and for an unselected, non-corrective group for the same period were compared. The same group already studied as to median scores in the speech tests (Table VII) was used.  The results are given in Table VIII.

TABLE VIII

Number of subjects in Speech Correction Group . . . 141
Number of subjects in Freshman Unselected Group . . . 130

Total . 271

| Median Scores | Speech Correction Group | Control Group |
|---|---|---|
| Scholastic Aptitude Test (Psychological) . | 532 | 524 |
| Range of scores . . . . . | 365–736 | 349–725 |
| Scholarship average . . . . | 79·8 | 78·6 |
| Range of scores . . . . | 62·4 to 93·2 | 66·2 to 91·6 |

This shows that there is a close correspondence between the average scholarship scores for the corrective group and for the unselected or control group. It is possible that had a carefully selected group of students with excellent speech standing been chosen, there might have been a wider range of difference shown in scholarship and in intelligence, but we believe after some years of investigation, correlations for different years and for periods of several years as above, that in college groups we find just as many students of superior or above average scholarship and of good mental ability in the speech corrective group, as of inferior standing. This is borne out by an earlier study reported elsewhere, including a group of 153 students held for speech correction, years 1922-25.[1]

The earlier study showed that 32 per cent. of the girls held for speech correction were in the highest scholarship group; 52 per cent. were in the two lowest of the five groups, the remaining 16 per cent. being close to the mid-line in scholarship. But when the intelligence tests were studied, for these same students, it was found that there were as many girls of high standing in the intelligence tests, as of low standing, who had been placed in the speech corrective group.

The studies of scholarship and of psychological aptitude therefore seem to indicate from all groups studied during the ten years, that there is no important difference in mental endowment or in possibilities of scholastic attainment in the corrective group as compared with either a superior speech group or an unselected group of students in the same institution. There are indications, however, that there are frequent failures in college among the speech corrective students, many of which are believed to be due to personality difficulties, mental conflicts and maladjustment. While this does not show in a comparison which gives only the median, or average, we know that there have been some important personality difficulties in the speech corrective group, and that the

[1] Stinchfield, S. M., " Speech Defects as a Personnel Problem ", *Amer. Speech Jour.*, II, 3, Dec. 1926.

personality factor is important in improving the speech function. Studies of Personality are discussed in another part of this paper, in connection with the Thurstone Personality Schedule given to speech corrective groups and to an unselected or control group, years 1930 and 1931.

These findings are in agreement with those reported by McDowell [1] in regard to the standing of stutterers, both in psychological tests and in scholarship.[1]

With one exception, every stutterer held for speech correction in college during the ten-year period, has been a girl of above average mental ability on the basis of the scholastic aptitude tests and the standing in scholarship at the time when such studies were made by the writer. Those whose scholarship has been below average have been found almost invariably in the oral inaccuracy group. The few girls with physical handicaps such as cleft-palate speech, speech due to deafness or following infantile or spastic paralysis, have been at least up to average in scholarship. Those who respond most readily to training are usually the girls of better mental ability and those who have good auditory discrimination so that they may check upon their own speech, even when absent from the instructor or the speech conference. The girls of poorer scholarship and those with poor auditory discrimination are those who have been held longest, generally, and who respond most slowly to corrective measures.

It seems to be important that educators should be aware of the presence and persistence of speech defects in girls of good mental equipment, and confute the all-too-prevalent impression that such girls are usually " dumbbells " or below average in intelligence, as we believe that our studies have shown that there are fully as many girls of above-average endowment as below-average in our college speech correction group, judging by a ten-year period of observation and study.

In the year 1923–24 a comparison was made between behaviour difficulties or personality indications of an

1 McDowell, Eliz. D., "Educa. and Emotional Adjustment of Stuttering Children ", T.C. Contributions to Education.

unfavourable type, and physical disorders or difficulties of the type which might interfere with speech effectiveness. The results are shown in the following table :—

TABLE IX [1]

Number tested, 340 subjects, including entire Freshman Class for year 1923–24

| | |
|---|---|
| Number listed as having personality or behaviour difficulties . . . . . . . . | 36 per cent. |
| Number listed for remedial physical handicaps . . | 21 per cent. |

This indicates that these students are well cared for on the physical side, but that the personality or adjustment problem is apparent in a larger number of students than are physical handicaps. It was felt that a further study of the physical condition of a corrective group as compared with a control group might be found to be significant. In the Fall of 1926 when other studies were being made, the speech correction group of 41 girls was compared with a superior speech group of 41 subjects.

The results are here given . . . . . Total, 82 subjects.

| Notations in Regard to Physical and Health Conditions [2] | Group I* Number of Students | Group III* |
|---|---|---|
| 1. Those having had from 2 to 4 of the common diseases of childhood . . . . | 12 | 12 |
| 2. Tonsils and adenoids removed . . . | 19 | 23 |
| 3. Subject to frequent colds . . . . | 11 | 6 |
| 4. Influenza, during or since the World War period . . . . . . | 15 | 12 |
| 5. Nasal obstruction . . . . . | 0 | 1 |
| 6. Enlarged glands or indications of goitre . | 6 | 7 |
| 7. Left-handed (as reported) . . . . | 1 | 0 |
| 8. Respiratory diseases such as tonsilitis, diphtheria, catarrh, bronchitis, pneumonia or hay fever . . . . | 16 | 14 |
| 9. Chronic pharyngitis or congested pharynx (at time of exam.) . . . . | 9 | 9 |
| 10. Subject to " fainting spells " . . . | 1 | 0 |
| 11. Very poor posture . . . . . | 3 (D grade) | 0 |
| 12. Infantile Paralysis . . . . . | 1 | 2 |
| 13. Weak heart . . . . . . | 1 | 0 |
| (Mean) Average | 7·3 | 6·6 |

The average for the corrective group showed a higher percentage of unfavourable physical conditions than were found in the control group. The chief differences are that respiratory diseases are somewhat more common to the

[1] Detailed report as to each type of difficulty has appeared elsewhere. Stinchfield, S. M., " The Speech of Five Hundred Freshman College Women ", *Jour. of Appl. Psychol.*, IX, No. 2, June 1925.

[2] By courtesy of the College Health Department.

* Group I, Corrective Group. Group III, Superior Speech Group.

corrective than to the control group. The control groups report more attention to diseased adenoids and tonsils, and this fact may account for the better speech hygiene in the one group as compared with the other, the corrective group. The corrective group is subject to more frequent colds and influenza than is the control group. The poor posture found in the corrective group has been checked with a later study which appears in this chapter, and the results are very similar for the two groups studied during two separate years and with a different set of girls.

## Respiration

During the year 1926–27, a careful record was kept of the scores made by using the Spaulding Wet Spirometer, as a rough check on respiration in the speech corrective group. The subjects number 27, or the entire corrective group then working with the writer. The results were compared with the norms for a superior speech group, and with Smedley's Norms for Vital Capacity.

SCORES ON RESPIRATION. SPEECH CORRECTIVE GROUP, 27 SUBJECTS
Compared with Superior Speech Group and with Smedley's
Norms for Vital Capacity, 1926–27

|  | Corrective Speech Group | Average Score (Mean) Superior Speech Group |
|---|---|---|
| Quiet respiration . . . . | 392 c.c. | 500 c.c. |
| Respiration preparatory to speaking . | 514 c.c. | 750 c.c. |
| Vital capacity . . . . . | 2083 | Smedley's norms = 2266 (16 yrs.) to 2343 (18 yrs.) |

It is evident from the above that even making a rough estimate, which depends somewhat upon the type of spirometer used, and allowing for some variations, the girls in the speech-corrective group fall below the average for a better speech group in quiet respiration and in preparation for speech such as would naturally call for greater volume of air. Also the vital capacity falls below Smedley's norms both for sixteen- and for eighteen-year-old girls.

Studies in respiration made in the department of physiology, including 1337 Mount Holyoke College students,

1925 to 1929 inclusive,[1] in which the Collins Spirometer was used, show that the average for our college freshmen is at least 3000 c.c. For the number studied it was actually 3280. Even allowing for variations in the Collins Spirometer used in the department of physiology and the Spalding Wet Spirometer used in the psychology department, the figures for the corrective speech group are low on vital capacity as compared with either Smedley's norms or the later norms found in the Mount Holyoke study.[2]

While the department of physiology found a difference in academic standing which favoured the high-vital-capacity group when compared with those of low vital capacity, they found that the chief difference seemed to be in participation in active exercise, extra-curricular activities, working for " honours ", athletic prowess, and the like. We find a similar factor at work in the corrective as compared with a superior speech group, viz. : that the girl in corrective work seems to have participated in fewer enterprises which favour growth of skill in speech, as compared with the girl from the superior speech group. She is less confident, socially more timid, more passive and less inclined to take the initiative, than is the girl in the superior speech group.

That speech training fosters the growth of power and achievement along these lines, however, is evident from the fact that from the corrective speech group have come a certain number of outstanding girls. Such girls have become leaders as much through participation in activities calling for speech skill and development of self-confidence, as through any other single factor, we believe, both from their own testimony and from observation of the development of these girls over a four-year period. We have had dramatic club chairmen, a chairman of the riding club, a community chairman, several members and officers of the dramatic club, house chairmen, girls who have contributed

[1] Turner, Abby H., " Vital Capacity in College Women ", *Arch. of Intern. Med.*, Dec. 1930, Vol 46, pp. 930–37.

[2] *Ibid.*, " A Study of Students with High and Low Vital Capacity ", pp. 938–945.

to the college literary magazine, members of college judicial board, and creative writers in poetry and dramatics, who were in the corrective group in Freshman year.

Shallow breathing, apathetic-inert responses based on poor muscle-tonus and lack of vigour, play an important part in the colourless, ineffective speech of many adolescent girls. Many of these are held for speech correction even though they neither " lisp " nor " stutter ".

Definite speech training to overcome these tendencies favours improved muscle tonus, is co-ordinated with the work in physical education, increases the vigour of the student, and favours a more harmonious and well-rounded development. Even the voice of a girl changes considerably in maturity and quality, under training, as she matures physically. But some voices fail to mature and remain at an " infantile level " in quality and expressiveness, unless definite speech training is received. It is a difficult thing to change the fundamental quality of the speaking voice in late adolescence. Differences due to individual backgrounds, ear-training, auditory discrimination, social discrimination and personal qualities make diagnosis difficult at the outset, but surprising changes are sometimes brought about even in the most difficult cases of infantile personality, immaturity of judgment, poor background and other unfavourable factors, as the college atmosphere often favours unfolding of personality more than does the home environment.

We believe that speech training is a matter of vital importance to every college man and woman, and we think that its omission from the programme results in serious and far-reaching consequences to the individual and to those in whose service he or she is later employed. In the Fall of 1931 the corrective group of 25 Freshmen and 5 upperclassmen was studied in relation to posture.[1]

Although the median and highest frequency for this group was B—the range was from B down to D and there were 12 girls out of the 27 whose scores ranged between D and C plus. The physical examiner reported

[1] By courtesy of the Department of Physical Education.

that in this group there seemed to be an undue amount of tenseness, limited flexibility, and poor postural tension, as compared with the findings for the average college girl. This seems rather important to the teacher of speech, as exercises bearing on posture, relaxation, flexibility and the like have not perhaps been given due regard in speech training. It would seem important that such exercises be included in working with a group of this type. It has long been part of the stock-in-trade of the actor and opera singer, and perhaps we have been too emphatic in condemning some of the methods formerly used with excellent effect in voice and speech training. In our emphasis upon the physiological and technical, it may be that we sometimes overlook the psychic side, factors of personality, mental adjustment and freedom or ease in speech situations, such as may be secured through a mental, rather than through an entirely physical adjustment.

Reports from the medical examiner on the speech correction group [1] in the Fall of 1931, show that in a group of 25 girls held for speech correction out of that year's Freshman class, 56 per cent. or 14 girls in the group are listed for some difficulty of the following type :—

> Malocclusion ; poor dentition ;
> Hypertrophied tonsils ;
> Unfavourable heart condition ;
> Deviated septum ;
> Low blood count ;
> Thyroid condition ;
> Menstrual irregularity ;
> Poor hearing.

This indicates that the speech worker should co-operate with the workers in individual or special physical education and health, for the benefit of the student, and in order to work in harmony with the Health Department in regard to the correction of difficulties in which the speech training may aid the student both on the physiological and on the psychic adjustment side.

[1] By courtesy of the Health Department, Mount Holyoke College.

RESULTS OF SPEECH TESTING, 1922–1931

ANALYSIS OF SPEECH TESTS AND MEASUREMENTS

CLASSIFICATION I

SPEECH CORRECTION GROUPS

This arrangement is according to the terms recommended in the Dictionary dealing with Disorders of Speech, prepared for the American Society for the Study of Disorders of Speech.[1]

Classification of students for the years 1922–1931 inclusive.

Number of students held for speech correction, 382

Total number of years, 10

| Name | Type | No. of Students | Per cent. of Speech Corrective Groups | Per cent. of all Students |
|---|---|---|---|---|
| I. DYSARTHRIA | Cases due to infantile paralysis . . | 3 | ·78 | ·10 |
| II. DYSLALIA . | Cases associated with deafness . . | 5 | 1·30 | ·17 |
| | Cases with foreign accent | 42 | 10·99 | 1·46 |
| | Cases with provincial or local accent . . | 7 | 1·83 | ·24 |
| | Cleft-palate speech . | 1 | ·28 | ·03 |
| | Oral inaccuracy and Letter Substitution . | 145 | 38·0 | 5·1 |
| | Lisping . . . | 77 | 20·1 | 2·68 |
| III. DYSLOGIA (due to psychoses) . . | | o | — | — |
| Three cases of marked maladjustment occurred in corrective groups at various times, but speech deterioration or dissociation did not occur, although in these cases the habitual speech was so poor as to place these girls in the corrective group. The speech and personnel workers were able to assist these students in making a satisfactory adjustment. | | | | |
| IV. DYSPHASIA. (Impairment of language due to weakened mental imagery, as in word - blindness, word - deafness, aphasia, alexia, etc.) . . . | | o | — | — |
| V. DYSPHEMIA . | Due to stuttering . | 36 | 9·42 | 1·25 |
| VI. DYSPHONIA . | Defects of voice . . | 65 | 17·02 | 2·27 |
| VII. DYSRHYTHMIA | Due to cluttered speech | 1 | ·28 | ·03 |
| | Totals . . | 382 | 100·00 | 13·33* |

[1] Robbins-Stinchfield, *A Dictionary of Terms dealing with Disorders of Speech*, 1931, private printing.

* 382 or total number in corrective groups, is 13·33 per cent. of 2864, the total number of students tested in ten years.

## CLASSIFICATION II [1]

### SPEECH CORRECTIVE GROUPS, YEARS 1922–1931 INCLUSIVE

Number of students, 382
Number of years represented, 10

| | | | Total No. of Cases in Speech Correction Groups | Total Per cent. of 382 Students (in Speech Correction) | Per cent. of all Students Tested or 2864 |
|---|---|---|---|---|---|
| | Stutterers (and Clutterers) . | | 37 | 9·68 | 1·28 |
| Articulatory Defects | | Structural . . . . | — | — | — |
| | | Paralytic . . . . | 3 | ·78 | ·10 |
| | Func- tional | Oral Inactivity . . . | 145 | 38·00 | 5·10 |
| | | Sound Substitution (including lisping) . . . . | 77 | 20·15 | 2·68 |
| | | Dialectic (local and foreign) . | 49 | 12·82 | 1·70 |
| Defects of Voice | | Structural (cleft-palate speech) | 1 | ·26 | ·03 |
| | | Functional (defects of voice) . | 65 | 17·01 | 2·27 |
| | | Paralytic . . . . | — | — | — |
| | Aphasia . . . . | | — | — | — |
| | Hard-of-hearing . . . | | 5 | 1·30 | ·17 |
| | Totals . . | | 382 | 100·00 | 13·33* |

[1] This arrangement is made in order that our statistics may be compared with the classification used by the White House Conference Committee in its report compiled in 1931 and 1932.

* 13·33 per cent. of total number (2864) is 382 or the number of students held for speech corrective work, out of all classes for the entire ten-year period.

## CLASSIFICATION III

Briefer summary showing types of difficulty for which students
were placed in speech correction groups, years 1922–1931

| | Per cent. of Corrective Group | Per cent. of all Students |
|---|---|---|
| Oral inaccuracy, letter substitution, and in-effective speech generally . . . . | 38 | 5·1 |
| Lisping (chiefly s and z sounds) . . . | 20 | 2·68 |
| Vocal defect, nasality, hoarseness, harshness, etc. | 17 | 2·27 |
| Stuttering (cluttering, hesitation and inhibited speech) . . . . . . . | 10 | 1·28 |
| Miscellaneous (deafness, infantile paralysis, cleft-palate speech, foreign or provincial accent, etc.) . . . . . . . | 15 | 2·00 |
| Totals . | 100 | 13·33 |

The column totalling 100 per cent. equals the percentage of
students who were held for corrective work, or 382 students in
10 years. The column totalling 13·33 per cent. represents the
percentage held for speech correction, out of the entire student
body examined, or 2864 students tested in 10 years.

These classifications show that out of a student body of
approximately 3000 students tested for the entire period, there
were 13·33 per cent. of the number placed in speech correction
groups during the ten years. Although a larger percentage was
held for such work during the first years of the giving of the
speech tests, when the average percentage held for such work
was 16 per cent. of the Freshman classes, years 1922–25, of late
years there has been some improvement in the speech status as
a whole, as is evident from the fact that the percentage held
years 1926–1931 has averaged 11 per cent. or considerably less
than during the earlier years. The average for all the years,
however, is 13·33 per cent. of the total number of students tested.

The reduction in the number held is believed to be due to
the slight improvement in the speech status of Freshmen ; to
the knowledge that such tests are required, and that speech work
is compulsory ; also due to the fact that an increasing number
of preparatory schools are placing an emphasis upon speech and
personality development as a part of the secondary school programme. The more such speech work is incorporated into the
regular school programme, the better will be the speech of the
student by the time he is ready for college, according to these
findings.

GROUPING ACCORDING TO SPEECH TESTS GIVEN AT
MOUNT HOLYOKE COLLEGE TO ALL ENTERING
STUDENTS, FOR TEN YEARS, SEPTEMBER 1922–1931,
INCLUSIVE.

TABLE I

Showing percentage of students in each speech group, 1922–25 (4 years)
when students with superior speech were excused from speech
requirement.

| Groups | Year 1922 Per cent. | Year 1923 Per cent. | Year 1924 Per cent. | Year 1925 Per cent. | Aver. of Total | No. Students | Year |
|---|---|---|---|---|---|---|---|
| I. . . | 18 | 16 | 16 | 16 | 16 | 220 | 1922 |
| II. . . | 19 | 24 | 44 | 29 | 30 | 350 | 1923 |
| III. . . | 35 | 42 | 29 | 41 | 37 | 308 | 1924 |
| IV. . . | 28 | 18 | 11 | 14 | 17 | 283 | 1925 |
| Total . | 100 | 100 | 100 | 100 | 100 | 1161 | |

*Key to Grouping.*

Group  I. Required Freshman Corrective work (Psychology Dept.).
Group  II. Required Sophomore Speech Course (Speech Dept.).
Group III. Satisfactory ; excused from speech requirement.
Group IV. Superior in speech ; advised to elect courses.

In the next table are shown the percentages of students in each
group when all students are held for some speech requirement,
with the exception of a few upperclassmen entering with advanced
standing in speech.

TABLE II

Showing speech grouping for the years 1926–1931, inclusive (6 years)
Total number of students, 1703

| Group | 1926 Per cent. | 1927 Per cent. | 1928 Per cent. | 1929 Per cent. | 1930 Per cent. | 1931 Per cent. | Aver. of Total | No. Students | Year |
|---|---|---|---|---|---|---|---|---|---|
| I. . . | 19 | 11 | 9 | 11 | 10 | 9 | 11 | 257 | 1926 |
| II. . . | 28 | 46 | 46 | 41 | 46 | 49 | 43 | 295 | 1927 |
| III. . . | 48 | 40 | 43 | 46 | 43.6 | 39 | 43 | 310 | 1928 |
| IV. . . | 5 | 3 | 2 | 2 | .4 | 3 | 3 | 290 | 1929 |
| | — | — | — | — | — | — | — | 260 | 1930 |
| | — | — | — | — | — | — | — | 291 | 1931 |
| Total . | 100 | 100 | 100 | 100 | 100 | 100 | 100 | 1703 | |

Total number of students tested, years 1922–1931, inclusive, 2864

*Key to above grouping,* 1926–31.

Group  I. Required corrective work.
Group  II. Required freshman speech classes.
Group III. The speech requirement may be deferred until Sophomore, Junior
or Senior year. (Speech is fairly good.)
Group IV. Advanced standing from other colleges, and excused from speech
requirement.

GRAPH I

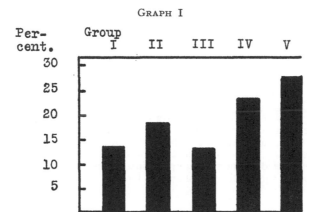

Showing scholarship distribution of 153 students in speech correction groups, 1922–25, Mount Holyoke College.

GRAPH II

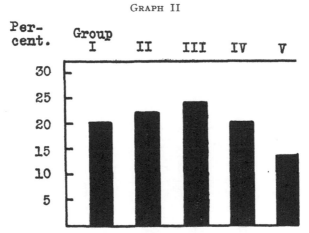

Showing distribution according to intelligence tests, of 153 students in speech correction, 1922–25.

### Interpretations of Graphs I and II

Graph I, showing distribution of students in speech correction, on the basis of scholarship, during the first semester of the Freshman year, in Freshman classes of 1922 to 1925 inclusive, shows that many of these girls are in the lower scholarship groups IV and V. Fewer of them are in the two highest scholarship groups

U

(I and II) than in the two lowest groups. There were 32 per cent. in the two highest groups in scholarship, but 52 per cent. in the two lowest groups, the remaining 16 per cent. being close to the mid-line. Something must have happened in the way of adjustment or methods of study, as these girls, according to indications given in their intelligence tests, do not fulfil the promise of the psychological entrance examinations nor of the college entrance board examinations, as we shall find when we compare Graphs I and II.

Graph II gives the distribution of the same girls, in the intelligence tests, and according to this graph it is evident that there are at least as many girls of high standing in intelligence, as of low standing. It is shown in the graph that more students were above the median for the group, in intelligence (Groups I and II) than below the median, as shown in Groups IV and V.

# CHAPTER XIII

## TYPICAL CASE HISTORIES

### TYPICAL EXAMPLES DRAWN FROM SPEECH HISTORIES

(FOR the use of the following material in its modified form, the writer is indebted to the Massachusetts State Department of Mental Diseases, Division of Mental Hygiene, in whose clinics the writer and her assistants have worked with children referred for individual speech conferences.)

### DYSPHEMIA

*Spasmophemia ; Speech Diagnosis of W.*

*Type : Stuttering. Also a Psychiatric Problem*

W. is a girl of approximately nine years of age. She walked and talked at fifteen months ; had two of the common childhood diseases during the pre-school years, with no apparent after effects of importance. Tonsilectomy was performed at four and a half years. No other surgical operations and no injuries reported. Family history regarding speech defect is negative. None of patient's early playmates stuttered.

School progress satisfactory ; home surroundings apparently excellent. Economic status good ; Protestant family. Stuttering increased at five years, when she entered school.

*Surrounding Personalities.*—Patient is an only child. Both parents alive and well. One grandparent lives with family ; family history negative so far as background for speech defect is concerned. Grandparent has not interfered with parents in the education of the child, it seems quite clear.

*The Child.*—Difficult, instrumental delivery at birth. Dentition delayed. History of delayed walking and talking. Born left-handed. No history of convulsions. Parents say she was " converted to right-handedness very easily ". Health has been normal, habits of sleeping and eating normal and undesirable habits denied.

*Intellectual Life.*—Mental age about three years in advance of chronological age. Started school at five years and has easily kept abreast of her class. Excellent memory above average. Intelligence. Speech defect interferes with school progress in oral work only. Tends to jump to conclusions without sufficient reasoning.

Play life is normal. Socially she seems well poised and alert, but is subject to temper tantrums. Rather " cocky " and inclined to show off, like many only children. Responsive to praise and suggestion. Has been pushed ahead in school, and this has not been the best thing for her, because of her speech defect.

*Onset of Speech Defect.*—Child was changed from left- to right-handedness in early infancy " without any speech disturbance ", the parents claim. The family spoke mostly German, and the child early began to speak both languages, so that by the time she was three years of age she had somewhat of a vocabulary in both. She spoke both until she entered school, after which time English was spoken exclusively. At four and a half years of age tonsilectomy was performed, and following recovery from the operation the child began to stutter and has stuttered ever since.

*Speech Diagnosis.*—The early developmental history, so far as speech development was concerned, was sufficiently unfavourable as to form a fruitful soil for the development of speech hesitation. In the first place, the handedness of the child, which was apparently indicative of right-cerebral dominance, was changed before the speech habits were well formed, and although no speech defect was immediately apparent, it is to be noted that a second feature enters into the picture at this point which adds to the unfavourable background. The child was forced to think and to speak in two languages from the outset. She might ordinarily have done this easily, as is the case with many children born in foreign countries where there is an intermixture of languages. But the interference with handedness, just at this time would seem to be a sufficient reason for interference with the motor speech habits, and would provide a sufficient explanation for the appearance of stuttering. There is, however, a third element which must be kept in mind. At about the age of three, also, the child was found to have a nasal obstruction, and both adenoids and tonsils were removed. Immediately following recovery from the operation the stuttering began to be apparent. This points towards the possibility of traumatic shock following the surgical operation, plus the factor of interference with motor speech habits, plus the necessity for thinking and expressing herself in two languages. Under these circumstances it is not surprising that a speech defect should appear.

*Treatment.*—During the school year the child came to the speech clinic once a week, receiving eighteen speech conferences in all. A final interview was given the mother by the speech worker, for guidance during the summer vacation. The child was referred twice during the year to the psychiatrist for additional guidance, because of certain factors in the home which were unfavourable. Psychiatrist's advice served to secure fuller co-operation within the home. School co-operation has always been good.

*Speech Tests.*—The score in Articulation Test on all English sounds was 84 out of a possible 100 points at the first lesson. Her score on the same test in January was 90 out of a possible 100 points, and her final score consisting of the ability to read and pronounce the sounds correctly aloud, and without stuttering, was 100 points when tested in May. At the outset she frequently stumbled on words beginning with *p, b, m, t, d, n, k, g, th, ch,* and *j, l* and *r, h* and *wh,* as well on the short vowel *i* at the beginning of sentences. She did not stutter uniformly on these sounds and her blocking sometimes occurred on other sound groups, but chiefly on these.

In Silent and Oral Reading she is above her grade norm, but her hesitation in speech interferes with her enjoyment of oral reading.

Her vocabulary is above average for grade.

During the speech conferences which varied in length from half to three-quarters of an hour, she was sometimes dealt with by herself and sometimes came with another girl of her age, also a stutterer, but whose personality was such that it was felt that the association between these two would be beneficial for both, at least part of the time. One was over-confident, the other deliberate, better poised, quieter in manner and disposition, but both working together to their mutual advantage.

At each conference they were allowed to give a résumé of whatever had interested them during the week, and were given suggestions and stimulating stories to read at home and to retell to the worker. They were asked to try to participate in the school work whenever they felt they would like to recite, and to try to reach the stage of actual participation in class work as soon as possible. The co-operation of the teacher was received, and both within a short time were responding favourably to suggestions and were able to read and to recite with much lessening of the speech hesitation,—often with no blocking at all, during a considerable period.

They were asked to do a certain amount of oral reading, sometimes separately and sometimes in concert, with or without the worker's help, and were gradually brought to the point of reading orally with no trace of speech hesitation. Improvement in spontaneous speech is generally slower than improvement in reading. This was the case with both of these children. One girl was precocious in development, the other had developed more slowly. The precocious girl was somewhat undersized, the average girl was up to her age and height norms in physical development, according to the Baldwin-Wood tables.

The right-handedness was apparently well established in the case under discussion and no attempt was made to change this, as such changes can be done only under controlled conditions, and the changing of an established " dominance " is still under discussion. Without such changes, however, and as a result of weekly training, suggestion, speech therapy, practice in reading and oral response, in indirect attention to posture, clearness in speech, volume of tone, exercises in rhythm and practice in self-expression, there was so noticeable an improvement in both girls during the year, that unless there is a relapse during the summer, it is believed that fortnightly conferences during the coming school year will be sufficient to establish permanently the new habits of speech, and that by the end of the coming school year there will be a fairly complete re-establishment of normal speech, free from hesitation or blocking.

### Speech Diagnosis of C.

### Type : Oral Inaccuracy and Letter Substitution

C. is a boy of eleven years, attending sixth grade in a parochial school. Birth was normal, but development was slow, and the child was bottle fed. " Difficult feeding ", incidence of children's diseases, and slow closing of the fontanelles suggest rickets in infancy. Tonsils and adenoids removed at four years of age. He has had fractured wrist, and is undersized at eleven years, but only five pounds under weight. Removal of tonsils did not bring improvement in speech, as had been expected, and the infantile speech habits have persisted to the eleventh year. Younger sister beginning to " imitate " this child is one reason why the mother believes that both should receive speech training. The speech of the younger child is not so defective as is the case with the boy, and it is believed, from the negative medical history secured for the younger child, that the factor of imitation is the primary cause of oral inaccuracy and letter substitution in the younger child. The elder child is of dull-normal intelligence, while the younger one is brighter and more adaptive.

*School Progress.*—He has repeated at least one grade in school. Younger child has also had to " repeat ", and mother believes that the older child is the brighter of the two. Some contradictions in the histories of both children as reported by mother. Worker has had to check the accuracy of statements by comparison from other sources. Language of the family is English.

*Surrounding Personalities.*—Father and mother living. The mother is subject to St. Vitus' Dance, with recurrences during several years of childhood; she is very nervous; had difficult labour in all pregnancies; and is frail of health.

Paternal and maternal grandparents : there are three dead, one living.

Other siblings : two girls ; both are older than patient.

*Economic Status.*—The father is of average earning ability and income.

*The Child.*—There is history of difficult birth, though born at full term. Food disturbances and loss of weight for some time following birth. Never talked normally. At age of four his speech was unintelligible. History of delayed speech ; he did not walk until two years of age. Defective dental development. Several factors in infancy suggestive of presence of rickets. Speech organs are normal, but malnutrition still apparent when child was diagnosed for speech defect at eleventh year. Ultra-violet-ray treatment was given and child began to show improvement. Also given cod-liver oil. He has narrow chest, round shoulders, and poor posture.

*Intellectual Life.*—His mental age is one and a half years below his chronological age. Interests normal ; somewhat dull in school work, and has had to repeat one grade.

Play life is normal ; he is good worker in home, obedient, quiet and liked by playmates.

*Onset of Speech Defect.*—Speech was delayed, and at four years of age was unintelligible, so that the speech has never been normal, according to history.  Growth history shows that there was delay in both walking and talking.  Rickets as a factor in the developmental history has been suggested as a possible cause for speech defect and delay in growth with consequent retardation.

*Speech Tests.*

1. Score in Articulation Test A (all sounds of English) 82 out of possible 100 points.  Deficient on about 18 sounds.

2. Score in Articulation Test B (consonant combinations) 50 out of possible 100 points.  Half the combinations were inaccurate or slurred.

3. Oral Reading Rate (Gray test) 108 words per minute, with many errors and mispronunciations.

4. Silent Reading (Starch test, No. 6) rate 190 words per minute, but with poor comprehension and short memory.

5. Of occasional speech inaccuracies, these varied from time to time, but he uniformly lisped on *s* and *z* sounds and had difficulty with *sh* or *zh* on all combinations containing *s, z, sh* or *zh*.  A sound similar to *r* was often given instead of *w* in initial, middle and final position.  *Y* was difficult, and final consonants were slurred very often or omitted in pronunciation.

*Treatment.*—Medical treatment had been undertaken successfully before speech work began, and the patient had responded well to ultra-violet-ray treatments and to cod-liver oil.  Speech treatment consisted of weekly practice for a period of five months, during which he attended the clinic eighteen times.  He missed some lessons through non-attendance.

Speech training consisted largely in phonetic drill, practice in reading simple exercises and trying to improve the retardation in reading as well as in speaking, as child was below reading standard for age and grade.  Progress in reading was slow, as time for this had to come out of the speech lesson and remedial reading was not a part of the usual clinical procedure.  Its need was apparent both in this and in several other cases referred, in which the children were found to be retarded in reading.

Improvement was checked and a record kept by the child in his individual notebook, which was a combination of exercises and of pictures used to secure speech responses, and some pages from Gates' *Round the World* Work Book for non-readers.  The child was given exercises consisting of simple words and sentences on which to practise at home, and if his progress warranted it, credit was given him in his notebook for sounds as they were corrected.  For apparent permanent correction a gold star was placed in his notebook.  Progress was slow, but encouraging.

STATISTICAL STUDIES

## BRIEF REPORT ON A TYPICAL SPEECH CLINIC
### (MASSACHUSETTS), OCTOBER TO JUNE 1931–32

| | |
|---|---|
| Number of children referred for speech diagnosis . . | 18 |
| Average attendance per clinic . . . . . . | 7.4 |
| Number of speech appointments given to all patients (during the school year) . . . . . . . | 209 |
| Number of times speech clinic was held . . . . | 29 |
| Final conference given to all mothers (entire session) . . | 1 |
| Smallest number of lessons given to any one child [1] . . | 1 |
| Number of assistants aiding speech worker [2] (regularly) . | 2 |
| Total number of assistants reporting during year (from Department of Psychology, Mount Holyoke College) . | 7 |

| | |
|---|---|
| Median chronological age represented in speech clinic . . . . . . . . | 9 yrs., 9½ mos. |
| Median mental age . . . . . | 8 yrs., 8½ mos. |
| Median I.Q.[3] . . . . . . . | 85 |
| Average retardation . . . . . | 1 year |

I.Q. status represents dull-normal, according to median and highest frequencies.

*Speech Diagnosis Summarized*, according to terminology of the American Society for the Study of Disorders of Speech, in order of frequency :

### I. DYSPHEMIA

| | Cases |
|---|---|
| Type : Spasmophemia (stuttering) . . | 10 |
| Stuttering with lateral lisp . . . | 1 |
| Stuttering with infantile lisping . . . | 1 |

### II. DYSLALIA

| | |
|---|---|
| Types : (a) Paralalia (lisping) . . . | 0 |
| (b) Letter substitution . . . | 3 |
| (c) Uranischolalia (cleft-palate speech) | 2 |

### III. DYSPHONIA

| | |
|---|---|
| Type : Rhinolalia (nasality) . . . | 1 |

| | |
|---|---|
| Total Cases . | 18 |

[1] Occasionally children were referred by the doctor or clinical worker for speech diagnosis, and these cases were not always speech problems, or it was felt that speech training was either unnecessary or unwise at that time.

[2] Assistants were psychology majors, trained in speech correction and psychology of speech.

[3] Compares favourably with findings of the White House Conference Committee.

## OCCUPATIONAL STATUS OF PARENTS

|  | Number |
|---|---|
| Group   I.—(professional)   .   .   .   .   . | o |
| Group   II.—(semi-professional) Managers, proprietors, etc. .   .   .   .   .   .   . | o |
| Group III.—Clerks, business assistants, etc.   .   . | 1 |
| Group IV.—(semi-skilled) Wire-workers, mill-workers, store-workers, porters, chauffeurs, etc. . | 9 |
| Group   V.—-Unskilled labourers   .   .   .   . | 2 |
| Total of fathers whose occupational status could be ascertained (2 out of work ; others either not living or unemployed)   .   .   .   .   .   . | 12 |

*Summary.*—Most of the above (75 per cent.) are from Group IV (semi-skilled workers). The remaining 25 per cent. are from Groups III or V (clerks, assistants, or unskilled labourers).

*Results.*—In the case of four stutterers, all facial tics, grimaces, habit spasms and inco-ordinate muscle movements have disappeared. The speech defect is arrested and has apparently disappeared. In order to guard against lapses during summer vacation these four are required to return for occasional speech conferences after the beginning of the Fall term of school.

In the case of three children referred for oral inaccuracy or letter substitution, considerable progress has been made, and improvement is noted in home and school ; but these children need to continue during another school year.

Two of the children, one a post-operative cleft-palatal case, and one a rhinolalia case, should go on, although considerable improvement has been made in both cases. They were referred rather late in the year and need to continue work until further speech progress is attained.

Four stutterers definitely need to continue work. There is considerable improvement in two, some improvement in the other two, but those referred latest need considerably more training. One will be referred to a summer school of speech, in all probability, as parents can easily afford special training while child is out of school, and it is felt to be advisable in this instance.

The remaining five have been either merely diagnosed or dropped for irregular attendance or lack of family co-operation.

Had the speech conferences been more frequent there is little doubt but that more absolute " cures " might have been effected. Estimating rather conservatively, we would say that 30 per cent. of the above cases might be completely dismissed, in all probability, without danger of relapse. The remaining 70 per cent. are in need of further training. Inasmuch as the clinic has been in operation from October to the first of June, with only one speech lesson per week, we feel that this is on the whole as good a gain as we might expect. By the end of the second half-year we should expect to dismiss another 30 per cent. ; but there are about 30 per cent. who may still need training for the full year.

# SUPPLEMENT

## SPEECH DIAGNOSTIC TESTS

(Reprinted by permission from *Speech Education in a Democracy*, Stinchfield, edited by W. Cable, Expression Co., Boston, 1932.)

## SPEECH TESTS AND THEIR USES

### I. Aims

In planning to use speech tests, it is necessary to have the objective clearly in mind. Is the test to be used merely to find out the size of vocabulary ? If so, a group test would be sufficient. Is the aim rather to give the instructor some idea as to the general effectiveness of the student's utterance and the types of errors commonly made, with the frequency of their occurrence, words slurred or mutilated, poor phrasing, unrhythmic utterance, letter substitutions and inaccuracies in articulation ? Are we interested in oral and silent reading and in spontaneous speech rate ?

### II. The Selection of Tests

All that the teacher may wish to know, is how many students are already superior in speech attainment, and who may be placed in advanced speech sections. In this case the interpretation of one or two selections from standard poetry or modern verse, anthologies and the like, including also a prose selection, would be sufficient.

If instead the object is to sort students into groups which shall separate the superior speakers from those of average proficiency, and to select for *special* training those who do not conform to a standard, then one must use not merely one test, but a team of tests which will give the examiner some idea as to the mental abilities of the speaker, the way his or her mind reacts in speech situations, and the types of speech difficulty present.

If standardized tests are to be used, it is necessary for the speech director to have a sufficient number of blanks or records prepared so that all students may be supplied with copies. The task is a lengthy one, for a single examiner, and since only one student can be tested at a time, it is wise to enlist trained students of speech or other teachers who can assist in the testing. In this way we may test several students at the same time, and may cover a large number in a relatively short period. Only an instructor with training in English Phonetics, for example, should be allowed to give the Articulation Tests involving all the sounds of English. An untrained tester too easily passes over many slight variations from standard diction. The poetry-reading test for interpretation should also be given by an instructor of experience in the field of speech.

There are a number of tests which are closely related to the speech function, which are of considerable diagnostic value, as shown by correlations obtained from certain tests, such as the Blanton-Stinchfield Speech Measurement series, which have been given to 3000 girls at Mount Holyoke College in a period of ten years. Some of these may be given by laboratory assistants, advanced students in speech and psychology, if they are specially trained for the work in a short preliminary training period.

### III. Practicability of Speech Tests

In order to conserve the time and energy of the teacher, for regular class work, the tests should come as early in the college or school year as possible. At Mount Holyoke College we utilize Freshman week for speech tests and physical examinations. Most of the speech testing is completed before college classes begin.

For the scientific sorting of students, the examiner should select a series from some of the groups of tests which have already been standardized. He may wish to use only one or two tests of a certain *age* level, to see whether or not a child conforms to certain standards of attainment for his age. Tests of linguistic ability, language attainment, language scales, reproduction of syllables and auditory memory span tests for words and digits are useful for this purpose.

It may be sufficient to give merely one or two tests without regard to their standardization. One or two brief tests, easily administered, may give the necessary information. The Articulation Tests (Blanton-Stinchfield Measurements) are frequently used for this purpose.

### IV. The Testing Programme

Speech tests, to be of most value, as a basis for follow-up work, corrective measures, advanced training and sectioning on the basis of speech proficiency, should be given at the beginning of the school or college year. Tests given at the end of the year may serve to show the *progress*, however.

Tests chosen should enable the examiner to classify his students into groups for training, according to the plan which best suits the school or college in question. A large city school, with limited space, cannot take many pupils into the speech class at a given time, nor can the teacher do the individual work which might be done in a smaller student body.

### V. Types of Tests

We present here a brief outline of various tests which have been standardized and used for the purpose of testing speech.

1. *Blanton-Stinchfield Speech Measurements*.

These tests offer a means for forming offhand subjective estimates of the individual's speech attainment in the elements of speech which may not readily be measured by laboratory analysis or by apparatus in the average speech group because of time and expense involved.

They also offer a series of objective measurements with weighted scores, making it possible to work out a numerical speech index when desired. A separate rating sheet is provided upon which to record the raw scores (when preferred), without other numerical computation. In this team of seven tests are included two Articulation Tests, A and B, Oral Reading, Silent Reading, Spontaneous Speech and Vocabulary. The tests are graded for pre-school and kindergarten use and through Grades I to VIII, with an additional test for college freshmen or high school students. This is called the Adult Test.

A series of pictures of objects is provided for the pre-school or kindergarten child, and for all subjects whose language is not advanced sufficiently to enable the child to take tests involving reading. A group of objects has also been arranged for children with whom the pictures cannot be used, such as blind children, children with retarded speech development, children of foreign birth, and the mentally defective child.

*Material.*—This is best illustrated by outlining the material used for a single school group.[1]

GRADE I.

Complete Speech Measurement Rating Sheet for No. I A.
Articulation Test Rating Test I A.
Eleven charts constituting Articulation Test I A.
(For pre-school, kindergarten and first three grades.)
Score Sheet for Articulation Test A.
Oral Reading Test I (Gray).
Silent Reading Test I (Starch).
Pictures I, II and III for Spontaneous Speech.
Vocabulary Test.

*Adult Test.*—Speech Questionnaire for high school or college students.

Articulation Test A and B, No. 5.
Complete Speech Measurement Rating Sheet for Nos. 2–5 (same as for Grades IV to VIII).
Articulation Test Rating Sheet for Nos. 2–5 (as for Grades IV to VIII).
Score Sheet for Articulation Test A and Test B.
Oral Reading Test (Whipple).
Silent Reading Test (Starch).
Vocabulary.

*Scoring.*—The Manual of Instructions gives norms and explains the method of giving the tests.[2]

---

[1] See B.-S. Speech Measurements, Manual, 46087     [2] *Ibid.*

*Norms.*—Norms obtained at Mount Holyoke College on Blanton-Stinchfield Measurements for years 1922–31 are given as well as those for an unselected university group at University of Wisconsin, and a selected group of students with speech difficulties, comprising about 150 students at the latter institution. Norms for about 250 school children in the Madison Wisconsin Schools are also given in the Manual of Instructions (see Grades I–VIII).

MOUNT HOLYOKE COLLEGE NORMS, 1922–1931
ON B.–S. SPEECH TESTS

NUMBER OF STUDENTS, 2864

Median Scores

| Test A | Test B | Oral Reading | Silent Reading | Spontaneous Speech Rate | Per cent. Relevant Words | Vocab. |
|--------|--------|--------------|----------------|-------------------------|--------------------------|--------|
| 96–97 | 98–100 | 170–190 (Whipple) 77281–A | 220–340 (Starch) No. 9 | 120–150 | 96 | 73–78 (Whipple Test) |

2. *Additional Speech Testing Material.*

Downey-Will-Temperament Tests.
Downey-Wagoner Test.

This includes :

(1) Test for Speed in Vocalizing.
(2) Freedom from Load.
(3) Flexibility and Volitional Perseveration.
(4) Motor Impulsion.
(5) Motor Inhibition.
(6) Care for Detail.
(7) Co-ordination of Impulses.
(8) Concentration.
(9) Nervous Instability.

*Scoring.*—This is described in a booklet furnished with the material, which may be obtained from the World Book Co., Yonkers-on-Hudson, N.Y.

*Norms.*—Temporary norms have been obtained for a group of 37 subjects and correlations have been found between the tests and the outcome of a parallel series of writing tests, by the method of rank differences, utilizing tentative norms and time records. The results are discussed in Downey's *Will Temperament and Its Testing*, World Book Co., 1923, pp. 229–243.

3. *McDowell Studies of the Educational and Emotional Adjustments of Stuttering Children.*[1]

*Material.*—In this study Mrs. McDowell has compared 61 stuttering children, selected from some 7000 pupils, with a similar

---

[1] McDowell, Elizabeth D., "Teachers' College Contributions to Educa.", No. 314, T.C., Columbia University. 1928.

number of normal children, in order to investigate the " psychological and mental " aspects of stuttering. The results, including comparisons with standardized norms are described in her volume. published by the Bureau of Publications, Columbia University.

Mrs. McDowell measured her groups with the following team of tests :

Pintner-Patterson Shorter Performance Tests.
Stanford Achievement Tests.
Woodworth-Matthews Questionnaire.
Woodworth-Cady Questionnaire.
Kent-Rosanoff Free Association Test.
Wood-Rowell Health and Growth Examination.
A special test devised for pronunciation of vowels and
consonants. (Arranged by the experimenter.)

In both kinds of tests—those chosen for investigating correspondence between mental and physical characteristics, and those for choosing groups equivalent in certain traits,—Mrs. McDowell found a " surprising amount of similarity between the stutterers and the controls ". Her findings indicate that in corrective work, procedure should emphasize eradication of neuropathic and psychopathic tendencies in individuals.

4. *West Diagnosis Charts.*

*Material.*—This is found in a clinical manual of Methods and Apparatus, published in mimeograph form by H. C. Netherwood Printing Co., Madison, Wis., 1926. It contains suggestions regarding the equipment of the speech laboratory, physical factors, speech tests, case histories, tests of emotion and of intelligence.

*Norms.*—These are given for a certain number of the tests, and others may be obtained from the author.[1] The handbook is especially useful to the directors of research laboratories wishing information in regard to clinical methods and procedure in speech work, suggesting also much valuable supplementary material, and giving sources. Case history outlines are included.

5. *Suggested Equipment for a Speech Correction Clinic.*

A condensed outline of clinical apparatus, methods, expense and sources from which material may be obtained is given on pp. 183–186 in a volume called *Speech Education*, compiled by Arthur W. Cable, President of the Western Association of Teachers of Speech.[2] In the same volume is an outline for the teacher of public speaking, which gives the speech analysis blank in use at University of Washington (pp. 83–87).

---

[1] West, Robert E., *Diagnosis of Disorders of Speech*, 1926.
[2] Cable, W. Arthur, *Speech Education, Cultural and Scientific.*

6. SCRIPTURE, E. W.

*Application of the Graphic Method to the Study of Speech and Song*, C. H. Stoelting Co., Chicago, Ill., No. 46565.

The *singing flame*, voice keys and other devices for the measurement of speech are described in this monograph which is of importance to the laboratory technician in the field of speech.

The results of the Scripture studies of the voices of stutterers is also given in his book, *Stuttering and Lisping*, Macmillan Co., N.Y., 1914. Scripture's technique and method is similar to that in use in the speech clinics in Germany at the time when such work was initiated, during the early years of this century.

Scripture's *Researches in Experimental Phonetics*, which appeared through Carnegie Institution, Washington, D.C., some years ago, is of interest to phoneticians, philologists, neurologists and clinical workers in speech or lalophoniatry, trained in laboratory method and in interpretation of graphic studies.

7. *University of Iowa Studies*. ORTON, TRAVIS, JASPER, *et al.*

*Material.*—Methods, results of researches, experimental technique particularly with relation to aphasia and stuttering, have been described by Orton and Travis in joint work done at the State University of Iowa Laboratories, in the Psychopathic Hospital. Important work with stutterers is being continued by Travis in connection with the *Cerebral Dominance* theory.[1]

TRAVIS, L. E.

*Material.*—Methods, results of research, theories and suggestions in regard to the pathology of speech. Travis, L. E., *Speech Pathology*, 1931.

*Technique.*—Travis has given a large number of tests of physiological and mental functions related to speech and to other cerebral activities, the descriptions and results of which have appeared in various numbers of the Archives of Neuro-psychiatry in the Iowa Studies in Psychology, in the Psycholog. Monograph Series, 1932, in the *Journal of Abnormal and Social Psychology*, Vol. XX, 2, July 1925, and *Journal of Experimental Psychology*, IX, 5, October 1928.

8. BLUEMEL, C. S.

*Material.*—This is described in Bluemel's recent volume on *Mental Aspects of Stammering*, published by Williams & Wilkins, Baltimore, 1930.

---

References :

[1] Orton, S. R., " Training the Left Handed ", *Hygeia*, Sept. 1927 pp. 451–454.

*Ibid.*, " Studies in Stuttering ", *Arch. Neurol. and Psychiatry*, Nov. 1927, pp. 671–672.

*Technique.*—The methods which have been found to be useful with a large number of children in speech clinics are described in detail with suggestive outlines for finding out the speech status of children and adults, and for speech therapy in the form of drill and exercises to be given in small groups or individually.

9. FLETCHER, J. M.

*Material.*—An outline of Fletcher's work, method and technique is found in his text, *The Problem of Stuttering*, published by Longmans, Green Co., N.Y., 1928.

Fletcher has done notable work with stutterers and has outlined a classification of speech defects. He has formed his diagnosis on the basis of experimental studies and tests given to a large number of students, and for description of material used, norms and method, the student is referred to his book.

10. METFESSEL, M. F., *Tests in Pitch*.

*Material.*—This is described in the author's " Study of Pitch Variations in Speech," Iowa-State University Thesis, University of Iowa Studies, Iowa City, 1927.

11. SCRIPTURE, M. K., *Speech Diagnosis*.

Mrs. M. K. Scripture has described her methods for diagnosing speech defects, methods of treatment and experimental data in a number of short studies from the Vanderbilt Clinic. Her Manual of Exercises for the Correction of Speech Disorders, arranged by Scripture-Jackson, gives suggestions as to speech therapy, correction of faulty articulation and enunciation, speech building, and etiology. This is published by F. A. Davis Co., Philadelphia, 1919.

VI. EDUCATIONAL SYSTEMS WHERE SPEECH TESTS ARE USED WITH A BRIEF DESCRIPTION OF METHODS

1. *California Speech Testing*.

*Material.*—Various speech tests are used in the California System, consisting of some standardized tests and some arranged by local teachers. In San Francisco such work was under the direction of Mrs. Mabel F. Gifford, Department of Pediatrics, California Medical School Speech Clinic, until she became State Director of Speech Correction. For references to her work, results, technique and the like, the student is referred to Mrs. M. F. Gifford, Dept. of Special Education, Division of Speech Correction, San Francisco, California.

Extensive work in speech testing with tabulation of results has been conducted by Miss Alice Chapin in the Los Angeles Schools. For description and method the student is referred to Miss Chapin, Director of Speech Correction, Los Angeles Public Schools.

Miss Edna Cotrel in the San Francisco Schools and Miss Sarah Barrows in the State Teachers' College, San Jose, have made contributions to the study of speech of the school child, through their local work. For studies on dialect and phonetics the student is referred to Miss Barrows' book, *The Teacher's Handbook of Phonetics*, Barrows-Cordts, published by Ginn & Co., Boston, 1926.

### 2. *Chicago Speech Testing.*

*Material.*—For description of testing material used in the Chicago Schools the student is referred to the Board of Education, City of Chicago, as considerable corrective work is done in this city, speech tests are used, speech centres established, with special work for re-education of children having a history of birth paralysis accompanied by speech difficulty.

### 3. *Detroit Speech Tests.*

*Material.*—A series of picture tests and sentences for testing grade school children, with sheets giving arrangement of consonants and vowels in the tests, has been published by the Detroit, Michigan, Public Schools, under direction of Clara B. Stoddard, Director of Speech Correction, Detroit Public Schools. These may be obtained upon application to the Board of Education, City of Detroit, or through Miss Stoddard personally.

These tests are valuable for public school work, where Articulation Tests only are desired. For norms and results consult Miss Stoddard.

### 4. *Minneapolis Public Schools, Speech Studies.*

*Material.*—Under the direction of May E. Byrne of the Minneapolis Public Schools a monograph has been prepared entitled *Speech Correction Monograph*, Minneapolis Public Schools, 1929, which is rather a method for correcting speech difficulties than speech tests, but we refer to it here because it offers some constructive suggestions in speech therapy for public school use. For information regarding same the student is referred to Miss Byrne, care of Board of Education, Minneapolis Public Schools, Minnesota.

### 5. *Philadelphia Public Schools : Speech Testing.*

*Material.*—Tests arranged by local speech supervisors as well as some standardized tests are given in the Philadelphia Schools. For information regarding sources of material, results obtained and follow-up work, the student is referred to Mrs. Davis, Director in Speech Correction, Philadelphia Schools, care of Board of Education, or to Dr. Gladys Ide, Director of Special Education, Philadelphia Public Schools.

### 6. *New York City Speech Studies.*

*Material.*—For description of material used, results and method, the student is referred to the Director of Speech Correction for New York City, Mrs. Letitia Raubicheck, 500 Park Avenue, Board of Education, New York City.

X

Recent legislation in the State of New York which includes provision for increasing speech work, and decreasing the teaching load of the present teachers of speech has raised the status of speech work throughout the State.

### 7. *Wisconsin Speech Tests.*

*Material.*—For description of material used in the State of Wisconsin, under direction of Miss Lavilla Ward, State Supervisor, the student is referred to the Department of Special Education, State House, Madison, Wisconsin. Miss Ward is in charge of the surveys and follow-up work in this field. Numerous speech surveys have been made in Wisconsin, the first being that made by Dr. Smiley Blanton.[1] The most recent study is that made for the White House Conference, under direction of West, Travis and Camp, results of which will appear in the proceedings of the White House Conference, held in November 1930.[2]

### VII. SPEECH TESTS USED IN CONNECTION WITH MENTAL TESTS

1. Various speech tests are given in the practice of mental testing, and manuals describing the technique, norms and methods are in print and easily obtainable. The student is especially referred to such tests of Language and Comprehension as are found in Terman's Manual, *Intelligence and Its Measurement*, Houghton-Mifflin Co., N.Y.

### 2. *Thorndike.*

The Thorndike Language Scales are published by Columbia University Press and offer valuable diagnostic methods for the teacher of speech.

### 3. *Merrill-Palmer Tests.*

These give a number of tests of language ability and may be obtained through C. H. Stoelting Co., Chicago. They are especially applicable to the pre-school child.

### 4. *Baldwin-Stecher.*

Speech tests given to children in the Iowa Child Welfare Station are described in the book by these authors, under title *The Psychology of the Pre-School Child*, Speech Tests, pp. 134–140.

---

[1] Blanton, S., " Speech Disorders as a Psychiatric Problem ", *Jour. of Oralism and Auralism*, 1–3, 1921.

Blanton, S. and M. G., " What is the Problem of Stuttering ? " *Jour. Abn. Psychol.*, 13, 303–313, 1919.

*Ibid.*, " The Medical Significance of the Disorders of Speech ", *Jour. Am. Med. Assn.*, 77, 375 ff., 1921.

[2] Prelim. Com. Reports of the White House Conference, 1930, pp. 314–321.

5. *Starch, D.*

Silent Reading Tests may be obtained from the author, in the Harvard School of Business Administration, Cambridge, Massachusetts, or from C. H. Stoelting Co., Chicago, Ill., in the Blanton-Stinchfield Testing Material.

6. *Gray Oral Reading Tests.*

These may be obtained from the Chicago University Press, or from C. H. Stoelting Co., Chicago, in connection with the Blanton-Stinchfield Speech Measurements. Norms and results are obtainable from the author, University of Chicago, School of Education.

7. *Whipple Tests of Linguistic Invention, and Sentence Building.*

Individual differences in creative ability, in linguistic invention and " literary imagination " are outlined and methods given in Whipple's text, *Manual of Mental and Physical Tests*, Warwick & York, Baltimore, 1910, pp. 435–445. A sufficient number of scores have been found to serve as temporary norms, and these are also included within this passage.

8. *Additional Mental Tests which are useful in testing Speech.*

*A.* Bronner, Healy, Lowe, Shimberg : *A Manual of Individual Mental Tests*, Little, Brown & Co., Boston, 1927 ; " Language and Ideational Tests ", pp. 29–63.

*B.* Thorndike, *Language Scales*, T.C.

*C.* Trabue, *Measure your Mind*, 1921.

*D.* Wells, " Linguistic Lapses ", *Archiv. of Philos., Psychol. and Scientific Method*, Sc. Press, N.Y., 6, June 1906. This gives the results obtained by Wells in using Nonsense Syllables for testing speech, and suggests a useful method for testing when one prefers to use meaningless material in order to better conceal the *test sound.*

*E.* Wells, F. L., *Mental Tests in Clinical Practice*. See " Personality Study ", pp. 263–277.

*F.* Haggerty, *Reading Tests*. These may be obtained from the author, University of Minnesota, or World Book Co., Yonkers, N.Y., publishers. There are two sets of tests in this series—one arranged for Grades I–II, and the second series for Grades III–IX.

*G.* Descœudres, Alice, *Tests in Power of Language*. This consists of a series of nine tests in which children are required to name objects in pictures shown them, two pictures having opposite attributes being used. The child must find the opposite attribute for himself ; the remaining tests consist of :

(1) Filling in missing words in easy omissions.
(2) Repetition of numbers pronounced to them.
(3) Naming six callings, as " Who sells tomatoes ? " etc.

(4) Naming six materials.
(5) Giving opposites from memory.
(6) Naming ten colours.
(7) Finding twelve verbs.
(8) Giving a list of twenty-five words of increasing difficulty.

In her discussion of norms Miss Descœudres distinguishes between children of labouring and of professional families, showing some social differences in the quality of the word responses given.[1]

*H.* Miscellaneous.

Visual and Auditory Acuity Tests, C. H. Stoelting & Co., Chicago.

Diagnostic Reading Examination, Monroe, Stoelting & Co.

Phono-Projectoscope, Metfessel and Tiffin, *ibid.*

Seashore Audiometer, *ibid.*

Personal Data Sheet, Woodworth and Cady, *ibid.*

Woodworth-Wells Questionnaire, *ibid.*

Thurstone Personality Inventory, University of Chicago Press, Ill.

Recreational Interview, Wannamaker's, C. H. Stoelting & Co.

Occupational Inventory, Simpson, *ibid.*

West's Armamentarium for speech diagnosis, *ibid.*

Phonographic Records made by G. Bernard Shaw, Lloyd James, Daniel Jones, *et al*, Linguaphone Institute, London.

Phonographic Reproducing Arm, Ogden, Linguaphone Institute.

Gadget for testing oral and nasal air currents, MacLeod, King's College Hospital, London.

Model of Larynx (small, practical size), Sherman K. Smith, N.Y.

Vocal Apparatus Charts and accessory charts with movable parts, *ibid.*

---

[1] Stern, W., *Psychology of Early Childhood*, N.Y., 1924, pp. 174–184.

# INDEX

Abilities, 3
  adult, 7
  infant, 7
  linguistic, 7
Abnormality
  temperamental, 142
Accent, 17, 189, 201
Action, 10
Activities
  bi-manual, 230
Adenoids, 122
Adjustment
  social, 147
Age
  at onset of stuttering, 123
  chronological, 43, 71, 73
  median, in speech tests, 285
  mental, 13
Agitophemia, 27, 116, 117
Agrammalogia, 25, 141
Agraphia, 161
Alalia, 25, 35, 36, 43
  cophotica, 25
  mutism, 35
  organica, 25, 35
  physiologica, 25, 43
  prolongata, 25, 44
Alcoholism
  paralysis agitans in, 104
Alexia, 33, 87, 88, 161
Allport, G. W., and F. H., 215
Alogia, 25, 141
  absence of ideas, 25, 141
Alphabet
  manual of, 39
Ambidexterity, 222-238
American Society for the Study of
    Disorders of Speech, 24, 80,
    312
Amnesia, 31
  auditory, 31, 34, 113
  visual, 31, 34
  transient, 31, 34
  retrograde, 158
Anæmia
  cerebral, 94
Analysis, 144, 147
Anarthria, 24, 80, 108
  anarthrialogia, 141, 142

Anterior poliomyelitis (see infantile
    paralysis)
Anthropoids, 4
  chimpanzee, 4
  emotional language, 5
  vocabulary, 4-7
Aphasia (see dysphasia), 26, 36, 42,
    86-88, 96, 124, 125, 152-163,
    302
  aphasialogia, 141, 142
  articulatory, 36
  associative, 131
  auditory, 26
  functional, 131
  in infantile convulsions, 99
  in juvenile paresis, 98
  mixed, 26, 152, 161
  motor, 152
  nominal, 153
  semantic, 153
  sensory, 152
  syntactical, 158
  total, 26, 152, 161
  verbal, 153
  visual, 26, 88
  Wernicke's sensory, 153
Aphemia, 27, 36, 116, 119
  pathematica, 116
  plastica, 116
  spasmodica, 116
Aphonia, 27, 76, 112, 143, 187
  absence of voice, 27
  apophatica, 27
  hysterica, 27
  organica, 27
  paralytica, 27
  paranoica, 27
  pathematica, 27
    phonophobia, 27
  spastica, 27
  traumatica, 27
Aphthongia, 111
Apoplectic attacks
  in juvenile paresis, 97
Appearance, 197
  judgments based on, 197
Apraxia, 92
Aptitude (see scholastic)
Archiner, D., 114, 115

325